UNACCOUNTABLE

Praise for *Unaccountable*

"Every once in a while a book comes along that rocks the foundations of an established order that's seriously in need of being shaken. The modern American hospital is that establishment and *Unaccountable* is that book."
 —**Shannon Brownlee, author of** *Overtreated*

"A startling revelation of the dysfunction deeply embedded in the very culture of American medical practice, problems that health care reform scarcely begins to address."
 —**Peter Boyer, senior correspondent for** *Newsweek*

"A very readable, thought-provoking book that will be of interest to health-care consumers, providers, and legislators. The problems pointed out and the solutions suggested deserve to be part of a national discussion." —***Library Journal***

"This thought-provoking guide from a leader in the field is a must-read for M.D.s, and an eye-opener for the rest of us."
 —***Publishers Weekly***

"A searing insider's look at what really goes on behind the scenes at major hospitals and how implementing simple steps toward transparency can empower patients and dramatically improve the culture and safety of health care . . . A galvanizing book full of shocking truths about the current state of health care."
 —***Kirkus Reviews***

"Makary's book makes it perfectly clear that data transparency not only allows people to make informed decisions about their health but also nudges hospitals and physicians to be more vigilant and efficient." —***Booklist***

"*Unaccountable* is a comprehensive telling of multifaceted problems inherent in the current health care system—a book long overdue." —**David Olle,** *New York Journal of Books*

"This book should be read by all people, not just doctors and health administrators, so they can make wise decisions when it comes to choosing where, when and who will provide healthcare for themselves and their loved ones. You will be a wiser health consumer for reading this book."

—**Michael M.E. Johns, M.D., chancellor,**
Emory University

UNACCOUNTABLE

What Hospitals Won't Tell You
and How Transparency Can
Revolutionize Health Care

MARTY MAKARY, MD

BLOOMSBURY PRESS
NEW YORK • LONDON • NEW DELHI • SYDNEY

Published by Bloomsbury Press, New York
Bloomsbury is a trademark of Bloomsbury Publishing Plc

All papers used by Bloomsbury Press are natural, recyclable products made from wood grown in well-managed forests. The manufacturing processes conform to the environmental regulations of the country of origin.

LIBRARY OF CONGRESS CATALOGING-IN-PUBLICATION DATA

Makary, Marty.
Unaccountable : what hospitals won't tell you and how transparency can revolutionize health care / by Marty Makary.—1st U.S. ed.
p. cm.
Includes bibliographical references and index.
ISBN: 978-1-60819-836-8 (hardback)
1. Medical personnel and patient.   2. Patient education.   3. Health facilities—Public relations.   4. Medical errors.   5. Medical care—Quality control.   I. Title.
R727.4.M35 2012
610.7306'9—dc23
2012007740

First U.S. edition published by Bloomsbury Press in 2012
This paperback edition published in 2013

Paperback ISBN: 978-1-60819-838-2

3 5 7 9 10 8 6 4

Typeset by Westchester Book Group
Printed and bound in the U.S.A. by Thomson-Shore Inc., Dexter, Michigan

Bloomsbury books may be purchased for business or professional use. For information on bulk purchases please contact Macmillan Corporate and Premium Sales Department at specialmarkets@macmillan.com.

*Dedicated to my father, whose integrity and compassion
in the care of cancer patients have inspired me to be a doctor
and to share my story.*

Contents

Introduction

When I told my friends I was going to write this book, many of them warned me, "Your colleagues will hate you." But what happened was just the opposite. Doctor after doctor who read my manuscript told me that this story needs to be told.

At the center of this debate is a fast-growing movement of doctors pushing to make medicine less corporate and more personal. They refuse to keep secrets and they insist on being transparent about *every* option, risk, and mistake. The movement has no leader and no formal membership. But ours is a cause many health care professionals are as passionate about as the practice of medicine itself.

As a third-year medical student, I quit medical school in disillusionment—modern medicine seemed as dangerous and dishonest as it was miraculous and scrupulous. The crowning moment came when I saw a sweet old lady I cared a lot about die after a procedure she didn't need and didn't want. Her doctors had pressed her to do it. I expressed my concern to them that she really didn't want this procedure and was frightened by the picture her doctors painted of what would happen to her if she didn't go through with it. Despite my protests to senior colleagues that the patient was misinformed and wanted to decline the operation, surgeons persuaded her otherwise. They operated. She developed a tragic painful complication and died three months later. That was it.

I wound up leaving med school, telling my supervising doctors that the medical culture didn't feel right to me—it wasn't telling patients the truth. I enrolled in the Harvard School of Public Health, where I met doctors from around the world who were forming a new discipline in medicine: the science of measuring quality.

The foundation of this new academic initiative was an appreciation that the blockbuster growth of modern medicine had outpaced its ability to coordinate. Moreover, it had outpaced its ability to connect with patients. What I loved most about my new field of study was that I found myself among many students, doctors, and professors as upset about modern medicine's collateral damage as I was.

Ultimately, I found that I missed patient care and a year later decided to finish medical school. I then began a six-year residency training to become a cancer surgeon. My current job has afforded me the honor of entering deep into the lives of thousands of wonderful people, some of whose stories I share with their permission here. (In some cases, to protect their privacy, I have used aliases—as I also have for some doctors, for reasons that will be obvious.)

As a busy doctor, I have watched patients increasingly fed up with a fragmented health care system littered with perverse incentives. It's an industry that does not abide by the same principles of accountability for performance that govern other industries. Instead, our health care system leaves its customers walking in blind. All while simply rewarding doctors for doing more.

From my earliest days as a medical student I've wondered why the same patient wheeled off for heart bypass surgery in Houston might simply be given an aspirin in San Francisco. I have long considered it self-evident that good medicine is not location-specific; best practices are universal. Despite strong evidence that medical procedures should start with checklists, like those that pilots use before flying planes, most doctors did not use them, and to this day many still don't. Similarly, some notable hospitals choose not to staff their intensive care unit (ICU) at night with a doctor. Even more hazardous, a hospital can be well aware of its consistently high complication rate for a service it provides, yet have little or no incentive to do anything about it, leaving the public in the dark about its "danger zones." Without publicly available metrics of a hospital's outcomes, how can Americans choose where to go? The only thing most people have to compare is *parking*.

Medicine is competitive, but it is competing over all the wrong things. In the past few years, experts who gauge the quality of medical care have formalized fair and simple ways to measure how well patients do at individual hospitals. These statistics are telling; they identify the good and the bad outliers within a town or city. If you had access to this data, you'd know just where to find the best care in your area.

So why can't you get this information? Because Herculean efforts are made to make sure you can't. I was amazed when I first learned this. But then it hit me: A hospital is no longer the community pillar I knew growing up, with its altruistic mission guiding its decisions. Hospitals have merged and transformed into giant corporations with little accountability—and they like it that way. Patients are encouraged to think that the health care system is a well-oiled machine, competent and all-wise. It's not. It's actually more like the Wild West.

As a surgeon who has worked in some of the best medical centers in the nation, I can testify that American medicine is spectacular in many ways. Patients travel from all over the world to receive our state-of-the-art care. American research is the envy of the world. Yet this same medical system routinely leaves surgical sponges inside patients, amputates the wrong limbs, and tolerates the overdosing of children because of sloppy handwriting. In 2010, a Harvard study published in the prestigious *New England Journal of Medicine* reported a finding well-known to medical professionals: As many as 25 percent of all patients are harmed by medical mistakes.[1] What's even less known to the public is that over the past ten years, error rates have not come down, despite numerous efforts to make medical care safer. Medical mistakes are but one costly example of how health care's closed-door culture feeds complacency about its problems.

Years after completing my medical training, I encountered one of my favorite public health professors, Harvard surgeon Dr. Lucian Leape, at a national surgeons' conference. He opened the gathering's keynote speech by looking out over the audience of thousands and asking the doctors to "raise your hand if you know of a physician you work with who should not be practicing because he or she is dangerous."

Every hand went up.

Incredulous at this response, I took to asking the same question whenever I spoke at conferences. And I always got the same response. Every doctor knows about this problem—but few talk about it. Every day, people are injured or killed by a medical mistake that might have been prevented with a modicum of adherence to standardized guidelines. The silence about the problem has paralyzed efforts to address it—until now.

Medicine is its own culture. It has its own language, ethos, and code of justice. How a doctor approaches a patient's problem and whether he or she takes care of it or refers it to another more specialized doctor depends to a large extent on their institution's workplace culture. At some medical centers, profits are king, while at other places teamwork is a core value.

Doctors swear to do no harm. But on the job they soon absorb another unspoken rule: to overlook malpractice in their colleagues. Doctors are generally well intentioned, self-disciplined, and well trained. Most medical-school applicants would detest a career goal to overtreat patients or prescribe expensive interventions. But this is how doctors are socialized. We're subtly taught a bias toward treatment rather than restraint. And while we don't like to admit that the almighty dollar can influence our medical decisions, we all readily concede that it does—for *other* doctors. By my estimate, financial incentives lure the average doctor two to ten times a day, temptations that are not always ignored—particularly when treating patients with borderline indications, who comprise a large part of the patient population.

The gray zone of *when* to treat is clouded by a medical culture that favors action over patience. Doctors are rewarded for "doing something." Drug companies and device manufacturers sometimes give large kickbacks to doctors. This is rarely disclosed to patients, but it really ought to be. Hidden economic incentives behind treatment recommendations are turning American medical care into a hodgepodge of rigged, nonstandardized care.

Much of the wide variation in the quality of your medical care can be explained by culture—an institution's level of teamwork and its local sense of common mission. Culture is why a nurse at one hospital will, following orders, administer a medicine even though she believes it was ordered incorrectly, while at another hospital, a nurse will insistently page the ordering doctor for clarification.

Just as the financial crisis was incubated when unaccountable bank executives created a culture of rewarding short-term profits without wanting to know the ugly details about their mortgage-backed securities, so too does medicine's lack of accountability create an institutional culture that fosters overtreating and runaway costs. If you pay for health insurance or own a business, you know how this broken system is hitting your wallet. In both cultures—banking and medicine—nothing precisely illegal seems to have been done; just a lack of transparency that has allowed bad practices to go unchecked. Banks wrote their own rules, became unaccountable, and leveraged public risk for private profits. Hospitals have done the same: The only difference is that with hospitals, the bailout is perpetual. Now that everyone has gotten stuck with the bill, the public is demanding the information it needs.

The shocking truth is that some prestigious, large hospitals have four to five times the complication rates of other hospitals in the same city. And within good hospitals, pockets of poorly performing services abound. Transparency of hospital outcomes for common services would reward good performance, identify bad outliers, and drive improvement, harnessing the power of the free market as it should. We do harness the power of the market today, but mainly by erecting billboard ads and improving hospital parking. We can do better than that.

Discussion of health care reform is often hijacked by politicians talking in sound bites who like to oversimplify or misstate the point entirely. We all know the health care system is broken, burdening our families, businesses, and national debt. It needs common-sense reform. Transparency can empower consumers to make their hospitals accountable and make the practice of medicine more honest.

For every doctor who has called me a traitor for writing this book, five have thanked me. That's why I believe that transparency's time has come.

PART I
Some Random Doctor

CHAPTER 1

Dr. Hodad and the Raptor

"THAT PATIENT BELONGS TO HODAD," the senior surgical resident told me with a smirk.

It was my first day. I was beaming with delight. *I* was at the
greatest health care institution on earth—Harvard. I could hardly
believe people walking by thought I was a real doctor! I just wished
the packaging folds in my brand-new white coat weren't such a
giveaway of my rookie status.

Giddy with enthusiasm yet self-conscious, I masked my emo-
tions by adopting a serious, doctorly expression, keeping my eye-
brows militantly raised, and by speaking in a deep monotone. I
didn't want to seem defiant or breach any unwritten code. If I relaxed my face, I thought, even for a moment, my senior resident
might chastise me, saying, "Do you NOT CARE?"

I had no idea what I was doing that first week. Figuring that
out was harder than passing med-school exams. I'd trot after my
senior resident like a puppy, wondering—every time he dashed
off to check a lab on another floor or talk to a patient—if I was
supposed to be doing that too. Sometimes I'd just stand around
wondering, Did he forget about me? and When will he be back?

This happened fifty times a day. Finally I decided just to follow him everywhere—until I found myself tailing him into the
bathroom. I then tried to train my resident to command me to
"sit" by pointing a finger at my feet whenever he might be headed

somewhere I shouldn't follow. When he did remember to let me know, I'd stay vigilantly in place, my serious face screwed on tight.

As I acclimated to life in the hospital, the name Hodad constantly cropped up in physician circles. One day, hearing yet another Hodad reference, I felt I had to ask about this Hodad, as he seemed to be the hospital's most famous surgeon.

"Hodad?" I asked. "I haven't met that surgeon yet."

"Dr. Westchester . . . Dr. Westchester *is* Hodad. That's what the surgical residents call him." Another student, grinning, leaned over and whispered, "It stands for Hands of Death and Destruction—H-O-D-A-D."

I nodded sagely as if I knew what the heck she was talking about. Later, I asked another resident what it meant. He perked up, eager to relate his own personal story of how Dr. Westchester had come to be known as Hodad. A celebrity actor had once come to our hospital—"America's best!"—diagnosed with what looked like a hernia. He wanted an operation. Like many famous people who flew in from far away, he had specifically requested Dr. Westchester based on his outstanding public reputation.

The celebrity's condition was one of two possible diagnoses: a hernia that would require surgery, or a normal muscle bulge that requires no treatment. Hodad saw the patient but ignored the need to diagnose which he had. The famous celebrity walked into the hospital very much expecting an operation—so that was what Hodad intended to give him.

When Hodad opened the celebrity up in the operating room, sure enough, he had a muscle prominence called a diastasis—a normal finding that can mimic a hernia. Even as a med student, I knew a muscle diastasis didn't require surgery. But the patient got surgery anyway, as medically unjustified as injecting Botox into a furry dog.

A senior anesthesiologist had been called in to help with the VIP patient. The anesthesiologist hadn't assisted at this type of surgery in a long time. He accidentally made the anesthesia too light. Reacting to the pain, the patient suddenly began jerking around on the operating table before the operation was over. With one thrash of the upper body, the assistant heard a few dreaded popping sounds coming from inside the patient's belly. These were the sounds of the patient's internal stitches breaking, a scenario that surgeons refer to as a "hard landing." The celebrity patient was now at risk for more complications, from a surgery he never even needed in the first place.

Of course, like most of the patients I've seen thrashing in pain in the operating room, Mr. Celebrity wouldn't remember a thing thanks to the memory loss associated with the anesthetic—God's gift to protect doctors from lawyers.

His incision site soon became infected, but after a long recovery, he bounced back to normal life. And the result of all this bad judgment, bad surgical technique, and bad outcome? A massive outpouring of gratitude to Hodad and his staff, including a Rolex watch, flowers, offers of vacations, and plenty of hugs.

The resident who told me this story enjoyed telling it. It was as if it helped him cope with his stress as a battered surgical trainee. His pace accelerated as his tale unfolded. The nurses took pains not to ask Dr. Hodad any questions, he explained. Asking questions exposed them to the risk of engaging in some awkward exchanges with him. Instead, behind the scenes, they'd nicknamed his surgical-instrument tray "the wrecking balls."

The more I asked around, the more incredible the stories I heard about Hodad. It was shocking and amazing to me. How could such a person be allowed to freely roam the hospital? I wasn't sure whether I should laugh or cry.

It was only later that I came to see that Hodad embodied a much larger problem in medicine, one the public knew little about. I was at that point just perplexed and vaguely intrigued. The patients whose numbers came up with Dr. Hodad were just the unlucky victims of a system lacking in standardization, oversight, or ways to measure quality. And yet patients left Hodad's care—and the care of thousands of doctors like him, every day—overjoyed and deeply grateful for their shoddy treatment.

I got online and started researching Dr. Hodad. HealthGrades, an independent ratings agency, confirmed he graduated from medical school, was board certified in surgery, and gave him five stars.

Preparing to meet Hodad in the hospital for the first time, I wondered what he must look like. I imagined a modern-day Dr. Jekyll—disheveled, arrogant, visibly hazardous. Waiting for the demonic Hodad to turn up for morning rounds, I noticed a distinguished, well-dressed man in his sixties in an impeccable white coat gliding toward our group of residents. He had a debonair appearance that inspired supreme confidence. Seeing that I was the new guy on the team, he approached me first, holding my gaze with his eyes. Confusion overwhelmed me as I realized that this inspiring figure was the infamous Hodad.

"Good morning. I'm Dr. Bob Westchester," he said, leaning into me with a sparkling smile as I stood there paralyzed.

"Hands of Death and Destruction, my name is Marty," I thought to introduce myself, but had to choke off an urge to blurt out this moniker.

The truth is, Hodad was terrifyingly normal.

As we visited several patients together, I observed his compassionate bedside manner and warm demeanor. His patients absolutely *worshipped* him, clearly grateful to have him as their doctor. In time, even *I* grew to like him. He sat closely next to patients to comfort them. It was model doctor behavior that I still emulate and teach to my students to this day.

The patients were not to be blamed for their adoration. Behind his charm and soothing bedside manner, Hodad's patients didn't really know what was going on. They had no way of connecting their extended hospitalizations, excessive surgery time, or preventable complications with the bungling, amateurish, borderline malpractice moves we on the staff all witnessed. His patients chalked up their misfortunes to random God-decreed chance. Some would thank Hodad for saving them from a worse fate. What his patients loved was his commanding authority, his fancy title, his Ivy League stripes, and his loving touch. His patients liked his care, despite its infernally low quality in the operating room.

When it comes to medical judgment and overall doctoring, good listening skills are both a powerful diagnostic tool and have the power to heal. But watching Hodad in action made me realize that patient satisfaction was only half the story. Patients couldn't know what we staff in the operating room could see: that the man was dangerous, had poor judgment, and practiced outdated medicine.

Hodad's popularity was no aberration. Americans are brought up to respect and defer to doctors—a trust I, too, enjoy many times when I recommend a complex treatment to my patients.

The public's disgust with our broken health care system as a whole, however, is akin to its disgust with Congress. Americans say they hate Congress, and consistently give it very low approval ratings. Yet most simultaneously like their own member of Congress, saying their own representative is a terrific man or woman. And apparently, Americans like their doctors even more. A 2009 *New York Times*–CBS poll says a whopping 77 percent of Americans are satisfied with the quality of their care.[1]

Doctors work in a disjointed system with perverse incentives, little oversight, and a lot of haggling that goes on behind closed doors far from public view—kind of like Congress. Factors irrelevant to health care quality, such as parking, are the leading influence on patients in choice of health care. One day out of every two weeks, many of my colleagues and I travel to a suburb to see patients in a Johns Hopkins–satellite office park that has free and easy parking, addressing this paramount patient concern.

So how does a patient who hasn't been to medical school find the best care? The only real way to judge health care quality is to ask health care professionals who work closely with doctors daily.

Hodad's popularity with his patients was in stark contrast with the reputation of another surgeon on the staff. All the residents called him the Raptor. They feared him. Unlike Hodad, the Raptor fit the surgeon stereotype—six foot two, a relentless jock, able to lift a medium-sized resident off the ground with one hand effortlessly during his all-too-common fits of rage.

The Raptor terrorized patients and staff with his curt bedside manner and drill-sergeant humiliation of the residents. Hospital lore told of how he was approached by a would-be mugger one night while walking out of the hospital. The criminal, not knowing the Raptor, held him at knifepoint and demanded his wallet. The Raptor picked up the assailant by his hair, shook him down for everything he had, and threatened him in a deep voice before the criminal got ground traction and fled for his life.

I had the distinct misfortune of peering nervously into the Raptor's eyes several times during my rotation. It was terrifying. Crossing him in the hallway felt like a slow-motion Jurassic Park encounter between human and beast. My heart would beat loudly and my mind would scramble in preparation for whatever he might ask, whether it was the latest news on his patients or one of the many random inquiries he would come up with just to torture underlings like me.

"What was Ms. Smith's white-blood-cell count today?" he'd bark.

"Nine-point-five, SIR!" I would reply, praying for no follow-up questions. If I didn't get the information out quickly enough, I would brace for the Raptor's claws.

We were constantly adding new and more unbelievable chapters of how the Raptor offended patients. Our consolation prize for being collectively victimized by him was to swap stories in our moments of downtime. One intern was shaken to hear the Raptor, through a door, bellowing at a patient, "You are not listening!" and "You could die!" Once, the Raptor stuck a nurse with a needle—on purpose. He told her, You stick me, I stick you. Hospital legend held that he once broke the news to a family that their child did not survive by walking into the waiting room and blurting, "Guess who just died?"

The Raptor may have looked like a jock, but he was an odd character, no doubt about it. I heard he once ate food directly out of a patient's tray without asking, like a scavenging bigfoot, the patient staring on. At a medical conference in a nice hotel, the Raptor was reportedly seen looting an unattended maid's cart for home supplies. Rumor had it that on a short airplane trip he sat on the toilet for the entire flight, just to enjoy the extra legroom.

Attending surgeons often punished residents by ordering us to stay late after work or walk their patients individually—a tedious and dreaded task. When the Raptor was a resident, he once fulfilled this assignment by gathering his ailing patients to be walked for a group walk. In classic, efficient Raptor style, he asked each patient to report behind a starting line demarcated by tape on the floor.

One frail ninety-two-year-old Korean dignitary left the starting area with a few short, distinguished steps before all the other patients had gathered. The Raptor lassoed him back, yelling, "Get back! Behind the tape line until everyone is here!" The man stood there with his IV pole and ridiculous hospital gown in silence and humiliation. He later explained to the patient-relations representative, "The *way* that doctor walked me. I . . . felt . . . like . . . *DOG!*"

Not surprisingly, complaints at the patient-relations department abounded.

Patients simply hated the Raptor. His abrasive communication style offended about half of those in his care, and many would request another surgeon. They would sometimes ask to be switched to Hodad. This was especially ironic because, despite his awful behavior, the Raptor's surgical precision and insistence on perfection earned him a reputation within hospital walls as the best surgeon on the staff.

Known by all the other surgeons and staff for his superhuman surgical knowledge and gifted hands, the Raptor was one of our era's greatest master technicians in the operating room. His clinical judgment and surgical skill were impeccable, even though his beside manner was toxic.

To this day, the Raptor routinely performs some of the greatest technical operations in the country. He also continues to offend and emotionally injure patients each week. In fact, a few of the patients he has jarred have ended up in my office seeking a second opinion. I always ask what brought them to me, and the response is always about the same: "He seemed incompetent" or "He doesn't seem to know what he's doing." Of course, if only they asked the nurses, doctors, and technicians who work with him, they'd know that the high quality of the Raptor's operations is the envy of the worldwide surgical community.

I wondered how different life would be if Hodad understood his limits and the Raptor helped him out. They'd be a dream team. But it was rare for docs to work together when getting paid individually. Moreover, the hospital's culture didn't seem to encourage it. At most of the "reputable" hospitals at which I trained, quality was highly variable and teamwork notoriously lousy.

As an exercise, I routinely began asking patients why they decided to come to the hospital where I worked (Georgetown, Hopkins, D.C. General Hospital, Harvard, and others). Here's a sampling of patient responses:

- "Because you're close to home."
- "You guys treated my dad when he died X years ago."
- "I figured it must be good because you treated [famous person] here."
- "I figured it must be good because you have a helicopter here."
- "I figured it must be good because you do robotic surgery here."

Parking accessibility and parking complaints came up a lot. Other reasons included the friendliness of the reception desk (often composed of rotating volunteers), hospital advertising, and "I was born here"—hardly strong metrics of safe, quality medical care. In health care, unlike other service industries, satisfaction is only part of the story.

In my experience as a medical student, it became clear to me that patient satisfaction tells you something, but *where health care workers go for their own care tells you everything*. The only people really able to rate the safety and quality of other doctors are those who work with them. No one else really knows. During my Harvard rotations as a medical student, I asked the staff who they'd go to if they were dying and wanted comfort measures. They all specified Hodad, qualified with something like "as long as he doesn't operate on me." When I asked who they would go to for an operation, the answer was unanimously "the Raptor"—usually qualified with something like "even though he's a jerk."

The Dilemma of Knowing

During the Hodad-Raptor years of my training, I unexpectedly found myself on the horns of an ethical dilemma—I wanted to let patients know of the Raptor's technical genius and Hodad's incompetence. It's not like patients were shy of asking. They would inquire point-blank if Dr. Hodad was good. My way of staying out of trouble was to offer a carefully calibrated answer that did not speak ill of anyone. I learned this art form of double-talk from my senior residents, who were masters at it. It would become one of many new values modeled to me. I even noticed that my favorite professors kept the code of silence. When they were told about atrocious care at their hospital, they would refrain from comment, or on occasion express disgust, whispering under their breath— but never taking action.

There were other, more powerful ways I was "educated" on the code of silence. Once, in a hospital peer-review conference, I witnessed the futility of a brave doctor speaking up to condemn another doctor's careless decision to operate when the operation didn't meet criteria. The doctor at fault gave a justification that a courtroom would believe, but we all knew it was not true. It was a rare spectacle, yet nothing came out of it, except that the brave doctor who spoke up became a marked man. In a business in which reputation is everything, doctors who call out other doctors can become targeted by the practices they threaten. Suddenly, whistle-blower doctors notice they are assigned to more emergency calls, given fewer resources, or simply bad-mouthed and discredited in retaliation. Throughout my training I witnessed several doctors run out of town because their honesty and outspokenness began to poke the bear.

For me, I knew the ramifications if I sounded the alarm against Hodad—I'd be on the couch in the hospital chairman's office, a notorious scenario I'd been warned against risking if I ever wanted a job. In many ways, direct and indirect, I was taught that the code of silence was part of being a doctor. In fact, when I had time to break away from the chaos of the hospital, I'd pause and realize how far I'd come from my premed ideals.

As a student, I was often torn between the obligation I felt to speak up and the code of never bad-mouthing a colleague—much less a superior who would be grading me, as Hodad was. If only I had a way to speak up about doctors who were hazardous, outdated, or overambitious zealots. After one hellish on-call night, during a deep catnap I dreamed that I'd plastered a banner over the hospital's main entrance reading, DON'T COME IN! THERE ARE VERY DANGEROUS DOCTORS HERE. Though I never gathered the courage to openly criticize the system I encountered as a plebe equivalent, I did begin to privately tell my friends where to go for care, giving each hospital my own safety score.

If you want to know what doctor is good, ask hospital employees. The word on the street will trump a doctor's Ivy League degrees, prestigious hospital titles, and charm. Hospital employees know who one should go to, and who one should avoid.

A Pause before Hiring

Before becoming the chief of surgery at a prominent university hospital, Dr. Cee had earned accolades for having built an impressive trauma division from scratch. At one point, he was ready to hire an additional surgeon to join the practice. Dr. Cee met with his hospital administrators in order to begin the process of recruiting. After interviewing several candidates, one stood out: an extremely polite, well-dressed, and well-spoken woman with powerful credentials who impressed all the surgeons in the group. Dr. Cee met to discuss the candidate with his colleagues. They all looked at each other, smiling and knowing what the others were thinking—they loved this doc.

"Done," Dr. Cee said. That was easy; he had a consensus.

He then asked one of his administrators what he needed to do to get the surgeon on payroll and hooked up to a trauma pager. HR protocol required him to have one reference letter on file before extending an official offer letter. They all rolled their eyes, grumbling over the burdensome administrative hurdles to hire a person everyone wanted.

Dr. Cee knew the candidate's chairman, who had trained the recruit throughout residency and subspecialty training. Perfect. He'd knock this requirement out with an e-mail and get the recruit on board quickly.

Dr. Cee sent the recruit's boss a courteous e-mail:

Dear Distinguished Chairman,

It was our pleasure to interview your trainee, Dr. [Smith], for a surgeon position at our hospital. We very much enjoyed our time getting to know this highly accomplished individual, and we would appreciate your input concerning her technical ability, surgical skill, clinical judgment, and overall collegiality. We appreciate your input and look forward to the prospect of hiring your trainee.

Sincerely,
Dr. Cee

The recruit's boss replied promptly with a one-word e-mail response: "Run."

Dr. Cee and his colleagues were shocked—and relieved to have been warned. Curious, he asked other doctors who worked closely with this seemingly impeccable candidate. They all chimed in with grave warnings.

Dr. Cee's confidence deflated. He felt like a rookie recruiter from HR with no screening talent. To think that all of his partners were also fooled. It was a scary close call. A full day of interviews hadn't uncovered what everyone at the recruit's home institution knew: Despite her terrific manners and personality, she was a proto-Hodad. If a group of highly educated university surgeons could miss it after a day of multiple screening interviews, how could a patient ever know? The only way to uncover the truth was to ask the hospital employees who had actually worked with the person.

Teamwork as a Quality Indicator

Having worked at some of our nation's best hospitals, I can testify that nearly every hospital has a Hodad and a Raptor, with everything in between. I've witnessed heads of state, celebrities, CEOs, and other powerful elites demand to be operated on by bumbling Hodads without having the first clue that they were jeopardizing their health. I've also seen homeless patients operated on by skilled Raptors, totally unaware that they had just received the gift of state-of-the-art, top-quality surgery. Sometimes the odd couples of medicine combine their talents, if the bad doctors happen to know their limits and call for assistance when necessary. When teamwork is good, the hospitals have good outcomes. When it is poor, hospitals have worse outcomes.

CHAPTER 2

Danger Zones

A Tale of Two Polyps

As a surgical resident rotating through different hospital departments as a part of my curriculum, I trained with two doctors to learn how to do a colonoscopy. One was Dr. Cotman, a respected medical gastroenterologist. A well-known team player, he was very approachable and kindhearted. We nicknamed him the Rear Admiral—a name that made him laugh every time he heard it.

One day, during a colonoscopy we performed together on a patient, Dr. Cotman and I discovered a golf-ball-sized polyp that appeared benign. While Dr. Cotman wasn't very good at removing large polyps through the scope, he also had no shame in calling in another doctor who could do it safely. With the patient still asleep, a younger colleague from the room next door popped over and quickly lassoed the polyp with a wire snare passed through the scope—a device he jokingly called a nine iron. He took it out slick and fast—it was awesome. The patient woke up from his screening colonoscopy and was told that a large polyp was removed. The patient was elated.

Days later, I was assisting another doctor, Dr. Frederick, a respected colorectal surgeon, on an identical colonoscopy procedure. Just as with Dr. Cotman, this surgeon discovered a golf-ball-sized polyp. It looked so similar, it was almost as if it were the same patient. I asked the surgeon if he was going to remove it using the slick wire-snare technique. He replied, "I like to remove these in the operating room by taking out the colon," referring to a separately scheduled open operation to remove half of the colon through a large abdominal incision.

What?! I thought to myself. Why not just turn over the patient to the expert next door?

Remembering the last success I witnessed, surgery to remove the colon sounded like overkill to me. I told Dr. Frederick about how I'd seen a doctor remove a similar polyp with a snare and offered to call him. Dr. Frederick replied, "I just like to take these out with surgery."

The patient awoke from his screening colonoscopy and was told that a large polyp was discovered and that it would require a major operation at some point in the coming weeks. He was terrified. Weeks later the patient had his major operation and was told that the mass was benign.

It struck me that both the gastroenterologist and the surgeon approached the same problem totally differently, perhaps based on what they had been taught in their training. In doctor speak, we would say that they had different "styles." The only thing they had in common was that they reported to no one except their respective, information-deprived patients who, in good faith, trusted them. Everyone in the colonoscopy unit—nurses, anesthesiologists, technicians, me, and even the scheduler—knew this surgeon took disproportionately more screening-colonoscopy patients to surgery, whereas other doctors worked as a team to get the best doctor to remove polyps with a wire snare.

While nearly every employee knew this surgeon wasn't a team player—and wasn't really doing the right thing for many patients—their input didn't matter. It also didn't matter that every hospital employee respected Dr. Cotman because he knew his limits and listened to the input of his nurses—credentials that made him the go-to doctor if any staff member needed a colonoscopy.

To me, this was one of those moments that clarified how medicine was not a standardized science as I had envisioned it would be when I was a college student aspiring to be a doctor. The profes-

sion was much less omnicompetent or all-wise than I thought; instead it was largely unaccountable. What patients get can be
determined by whether their doctor can summon enough humility to always do what's in the patients' best interest. To this day, I
continue to see patients coming for a second opinion and am
shocked by the radically different care they receive for the identical
problem. (To this day, the gastroenterologist and surgeon described above—both widely sought after by patients—have thriv-
ing practices.)

How to Measure?

Based on my experience with seeing how doctors handle polyps,
and dozens of other medical conditions, I became convinced that
teamwork is a marker of good medical care. Later, as a health
policy researcher, I was eager to measure the phenomenon. I
called Dr. Bryan Sexton, a teamwork guru and author of a widely
used survey showing a strong correlation between airplane-crew
teamwork and pilot errors. A Ph.D. in social psychology, Dr. Sexton joined Johns Hopkins shortly after applying his survey to
improve safety at Continental Airlines. A warm, intelligent, for-
tysomething man and keen observer, Dr. Sexton is a master of
learning by listening, often with a smile as he strokes his light
beard. I found myself sharing things with this genuine and approachable researcher that normally I'd share only with my family. Bryan loves talking to people about their lives, uncovering
root causes and what makes them tick.

Our group brainstormed about how to use Dr. Sexton's methods to measure medical quality and detect bad outliers, i.e., hospitals littered with "danger zones." We noted the striking similarities
between airline cockpits and medical-procedure rooms: both
high-stakes environments with a formal hierarchy. Confidentiality was key to eliciting honest responses about workplace culture
and safety for both airplane-pilot crews and health care workers.

Dr. Sexton tailored the health care survey questions to specific
departments (or clinical areas) within a hospital:

- Is the teamwork good?
- Would you feel comfortable having your own care performed in the unit in which you work?
- Do people work well as a coordinated team?
- Do doctors and nurses do what's in the best interest of the patient?
- Is communication strong?
- Do you feel comfortable speaking up when you have a safety concern?

We set rules for the survey: At least 70 percent of hospital employees must complete it for the results to be statistically accurate, and obviously it must be anonymous so as to elicit honest answers. Based on employee responses, each hospital gets a teamwork score both for the hospital as a whole and for its individual departments and units. The above questions and other critical questions are used to calculate (on a scale of 0–100) a Teamwork Culture Score for a hospital, an Overall Safety Culture Score, and even a score for a specific unit within the hospital.

We began working on a study now known as the Hopkins Safety Culture Study. Sixty reputable U.S. hospitals administered the survey to all of their employees. Remarkably, we found that the safety culture among those sixty hospitals varied enormously.[1] Subsequent studies revealed that teamwork culture could also vary dramatically within a hospital (i.e., one hospital could have a perfect teamwork culture in surgery and an awful teamwork culture in ob-gyn).

The survey allowed us to measure the insider's perspective. It used the "word on the ground" principle for failing businesses: ask executives about the quality of service, and you'll get one answer; ask the workers on the ground, and you'll get the *real* answer.

Thanks to Dr. Sexton, we now had a clear-cut, scientifically valid way to measure hospital quality and safety from frontline providers themselves—the insider's perspective. Our research team asked the sixty participating hospitals if they would let us publish the results in the interests of research. They agreed, on condition that the individual hospital names would be kept anonymous.

Here's what we found:

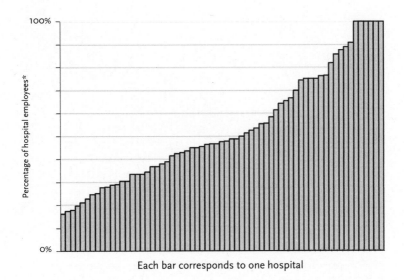

Each bar corresponds to one hospital

*Employees per hospital reporting well-coordinated teamwork at their workplace

Each bar represents one hospital. On the far-left side of the graph, we found hospitals where fewer than 20 percent of their employees reported good teamwork. Remarkably, at one third of the hospitals, a majority of the employees believed the teamwork was bad. Conversely, some hospitals on the right had an impressive 99 percent of their staffs reporting that their hospital had good teamwork. Participating hospitals began to tell us that their survey results also correlated to infection rates and patient outcomes at their hospitals. And most recently, our own research team has found similar correlations.

This makes sense. Imagine seeing a spread of teamwork culture like this for the hospitals in your town or city. Now imagine that within those hospitals, you could see the spread for obstetrics, surgery, pediatrics, or any other type of care you might seek. You might be at risk of being an informed health care consumer! Think about it: Would you want to go to a hospital where, say, *only*

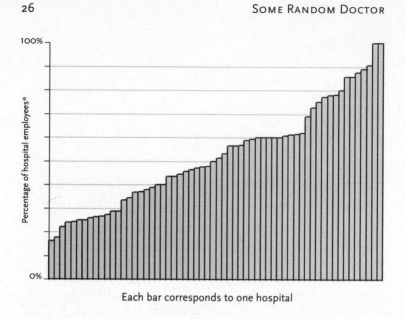

Each bar corresponds to one hospital

*Employees per hospital who would feel comfortable having their own care performed in the unit in which they work

18 percent of health care workers and employees report that the teamwork is good?

The survey also asked, *In the hospital in which you work, are your managers and administrators responsive to your patient-safety concerns?* The answer is revealing. At some hospitals only 19 percent of the hospital employees answered yes. At others, 99 percent of employees did. With every other hospital falling evenly in between. Trust me, I, my own family, and my friends are only going to hospitals where 90-plus percent said yes.

My favorite question is the simple safety question which, in my opinion, says it all: *Would you feel comfortable receiving medical care in the unit in which you work?* At over half the hospitals we surveyed, half of the health care workers said no. At other hospitals, as many as 99 percent said yes.

I'm convinced that the simple percentage of hospital employees who say *Yes, I would definitely go here for my own care* on the safety-culture survey is more telling than any *US News & World*

Report ranking, mortality score, or any other raw metric of quality care. Bottom line is, if 99 percent of frontline workers at a hospital would definitely go there, that would be enough for me.

At Continental Airlines, crews who described the cockpit as unsafe got targeted for an intervention in which pilots could talk about their safety concerns. Administrators listened to these concerns and addressed them. Soon enough, the airline's safety scores dramatically improved. Pilots also felt more valued, which probably helped to improve safety in itself.

If I knew the crew of an airplane I was boarding didn't think the plane was safe, I wouldn't get on the plane. Lives are just as much if not more at stake in health care. Unlike aviation, hundreds of thousands of lives are lost each year due to preventable mistakes by doctors.[2]

New Demand

Public demand to see the results of the safety-culture survey is growing. Who wouldn't want to know where to go for their care? The idea that good data exists but isn't viewable by the public is outrageous to many Americans—many doctors and nurses included. For the first time in history, Americans are demanding to have comprehensible ways to view medical quality. People are angry with being ping-ponged from doctor to doctor and from test to procedure, not knowing how to discern whether their care is of good quality. A new generation of doctors is also increasingly eager to level with them.

Even the federal government loves the survey. The government recommends that all medical centers use it, every year. Although the government hasn't made it mandatory for hospitals to publicly report safety-survey results, there's a free version of it on the Department of Health and Human Services' website at www .ahrq.gov/qual/patientsafetyculture.

The survey's popularity as a scientifically valid way to measure a medical center's quality and safety continues to surge. Hospitals all over the country, including my own, signed up to use it and find out how good their care was in the eyes of their employees. Hundreds of U.S. hospitals and many overseas now religiously conduct this survey every year. It is considered so effective, it can predict infection rates and other patient outcomes.[3]

Based on these findings, I asked the world's largest surgeons' association, the American College of Surgeons, along with the risk management firm Pascal Metrics, to partner with my team at Johns Hopkins to rigorously study the association between the safety-culture survey scores and surgical complications nationally. The correlation we found was striking. We found that hospitals that scored well on the staff survey had lower rates of surgical complications and other important patient outcomes.

Asking employees if they would go to their own hospital for their own care carries the power of sheer simplicity, especially when a survey can draw high participation from nurses. Nurses, after all, spend the most time with patients and with doctors. They take great personal pride in helping a limping man walk after a well-done hip replacement with few complications. But nurses can also be among the most angry and disgusted when they see one of their high-risk patients undergoing a dangerous procedure without the patient understanding what is being done. The teamwork survey gives nurses a voice with which to speak out about these matters.

Swiss Re, one of the world's largest insurance underwriters, was especially impressed by the Hopkins data on how simple survey questions of employees predict hospital risk, calling it the best-devised method to date.

A confidential survey encourages candor—data a face-to-face interview very likely won't elicit. And it's easy to fill out: one page (front and back), it takes about ten minutes to complete. Across any industry, business black belts agree that the way to fix a problem is to measure it first, and the results of these surveys can be amazingly informative.

While hundreds of U.S. hospitals now use the survey, all do so under the condition that the results remain top secret, used only for internal viewing by the government and hospital administrators at the participating centers. When hospitals make decisions to not staff their intensive care units (ICUs) with an ICU doctor on nights and weekends, that is a "danger zone" that the safety survey readily detects. Similarly, when doctors refuse to use a checklist before doing procedures, the survey yields a low safety-culture score among the staff. Yet hospitals have little or no incentive to make their safety scores public. Hospital competition is fierce, and millions of dollars in daily revenue are at stake if a reputation is tarnished by a low safety score. As a result of this suppression of data, a hospital's administrators are often the only ones to know of their hospital's low safety score, with little or no incentive to improve it. I am often bewildered at the ethics of a corporation that is aware of a dangerous product yet continues to sell it. Goldman Sachs and other investment banks were publicly admonished in a congressional hearing for selling investment products that they internally spoke of as bad deals and were betting against. How much more serious is the problem of hospitals actively selling services that they know are far more unsafe than the national average?

Transparency would bring on a shakeout, but the end result would be that hospitals that ranked low on the safety culture survey would quickly address their problems. While I sympathize with hospitals who feel threatened by transparency of safety-culture results, I sympathize more with misled patients. Hospitals now generate midsize corporate-level profits each year and spend millions in marketing. I have seen well-intended patients put themselves in the hands of hospitals with care that is substandard, even dangerous. Just as I can go online and see where Bill Gates or Warren Buffett are investing their money, the public should be able to see the data on hospital performance. It could spark a nationwide health care "spring," leading people to flock to the highest-quality hospitals in their area, while forcing poorly performing hospitals to clean house.

Much of the competition in health care shows up in advertising campaigns, money that might be better spent on more doctors and nurses or the equipment health care professionals need to do their best work. Rather than rewarding mavericks who choose to operate on every colon polyp found on a screening colonoscopy, better hospital management would focus more on quality measures, like promoting internal collaboration.

The survey is a powerful tool, but it's not the only one. To assess the quality of your medical care, you should also be able to look up a hospital's infection rate, the number of cases treated there, and its patient outcomes.

In short, data transparency, properly weighted, would empower patients to make informed decisions about where they should spend their health care dollar. If we had more of it, the accountability visited on hospitals would revolutionize the quality of medical care in every city in America, dramatically reshaping our health care landscape.

When my chief resident gave me the scoop on my rotation schedule at Arlington Hospital in Virginia, he called it a "machine." What he meant was that the hospital ran like a high-performance sports car, clean and faultless. This was no chop shop—our jargon for hospitals with a lot of "danger zones."

Surgical residents in Washington, D.C., might rotate through seven area hospitals for months at a time. After this kind of tour, you definitely know where to send your friends and family members for everything from a hip fracture to a mammogram. Those who work in operating rooms know more about hospital-safety practices and the frequency of surgery on the wrong body part than any hospital administrator. Contrary to popular opinion and hospital advertising, some machines are quiet community hospitals, and some highly trusted institutions are chop shops. Everyone who works there—nurses, techs, and even office staff—will know which is which.

A Principled Stand

Dr. Guy Clifton was one of the busiest neurosurgeons at Memorial Hermann—a leading Houston hospital. He was a distinguished chairman and a powerful figure there, yet he was growing increasingly frustrated by two trends in modern medicine: 1) hospital administration being increasingly removed from daily hospital care, and 2) modern medicine's growing appetite to overscreen, overdiagnose, and overtreat. To address these problems, he would frequently call upon his hospital's administrators to address the safety concerns of his staff. For example, as the practice of hand washing gained attention in health care, he noticed that there were not enough sinks for his staff to wash their hands in the ICU. Three times he had blueprints drawn to renovate the ICU and put in more sinks, but repeatedly his ideas were not funded by his administration. This despite the hospital making millions in profits each year. On another occasion, he pushed to digitize X-rays, arguing that digital access would decrease the number of X-rays that would need to be repeated. But, like most of his common-sense ideas, the request was ignored. His CFO told him there was no business case for digitizing the films.[4]

But there was one issue that Dr. Clifton was most passionate about fixing: the high medical complication rate he observed in the ICU. After looking into the problem closely and talking with the nurses there, he learned that bad outcomes were from "green" nurses learning the system. The ICU also had a high nurse turnover, which correlated with the high complication rate. Neurosurgical nursing requires specialized nurse training. Having to constantly reteach new nurses the ins and outs of the neurosurgical unit was a large part of the problem. Reinventing the wheel and learning from mistakes were occurring way too often. The staff knew about the problem and even brought it to Dr. Clifton's attention. The safety culture was poor, and the structure of the nursing coverage was a safety hazard blossoming more and more each day. In addition, Dr. Clifton noted how patients stayed in the ICU longer than they needed because of the teamwork issues there. Complications were high, and so was his frustration.

So Dr. Clifton devised a plan to restructure the ICU, which included hiring two full-time nurse educators to ensure continuity of care. Based on his conversations with his staff, he was so sure that the plan would decrease complications and lower costs, he guaranteed the department's administration that it would work, offering to pay out of his pocket if it didn't. In short, local wisdom guided a local solution that only he could figure out as he did. The request was put before his hospital administrator.

"Not a chance," his administrator told him.

The program never got funded and never happened. Frustrated with the resistance to his ideas and those generated by his colleagues on the front lines of care, he resigned.

The "business case" argument now made sense to him—and it was antithetical to his core values. He put the pieces together. He learned how the business of medicine works—the reason there was no business case for his plan to lower complications was that hospitals profit from bad medical care. He realized that hospitals get more money for each complication, X-ray, and extra patient day in the ICU. One well-known national study that was, ironically, released around the time of his departure estimated that a hospital gets paid $10,000 extra per surgical complication.[5]

Dr. Clifton's plan to deliver smarter care followed the trajectory of most common-sense innovations proposed by doctors and nurses: Everybody thinks it's a great idea except one group, hospital administration. Brilliant homegrown initiatives are often *not* acted upon by administrators because of the upfront cost.

Although Dr. Clifton resigned, he did not give up. Instead he decided to take the message to a broader audience. Passionate that Americans deserve better, he moved with his family from Houston to Washington, D.C., enrolled in a Robert Wood Johnson Health Policy Fellowship, worked on Capitol Hill, and dedicated his life to reforming health care in a nonpartisan way. The message was simple: financially rewarding bad medicine is endemic in American health care. He wrote a book titled *Flatlined: Resuscitating American Medicine*, outlining the perverse incentives of our health care system—a book I recommend to my students to this day. As a testament to what one doctor can do when he is willing to take a bold step, Dr. Clifton is having an impact on the national conversation on health care. Today, he lives in Washington, D.C., and works with both the military and private organizations to create networks of high-quality doctors. He is currently doing landmark work demonstrating that networks of high-quality care yield better outcomes and lower costs.

His principled departure from Memorial Hermann had a big impact there. The hospital lost millions of dollars in revenue from his absence. His cause there was later taken up by his colleague, neurosurgeon Dong Kim, who refused to serve as chief unless the administration delivered on Dr. Clifton's requests to fix the hospital's problems. The hospital's administration, in desperate need of a new leader to rescue the department, finally granted Dr. Kim his request. In a radical turnaround, the administrators listened to each safety concern and asked how they could fix it. A new ICU was built (with plenty of sinks for employees to wash their hands). The nursing care was reorganized, and new nurses were hired for the unit. The teamwork culture improved. Nurses wanted to work there again, and there was less turnover. Morale was markedly better, and postsurgical complications decreased. The average patient stay in the ICU was reduced safely. Patients' medical bills reflected the lower cost of safer care. Memorial Hermann is now considered by many in the field to be one of the top five neurosurgery centers in the United States.

CHAPTER 3

The New York Experiment

Transparent Medicine

ALL GREAT MOVEMENTS BEGIN WITH a spark. Just as Harriet Beecher Stowe's *Uncle Tom's Cabin* ignited the American abolitionist movement, the modern-day transparency movement got its spark from a radical experiment in New York.

At the center of the transparency experiment was Dr. Mark Chassin, a well-spoken, clean-shaven physician whose speech toggles from Harvard brainiac to street talk in the same sentence. Mark grew up in Queens and recalls how his father, a busy general surgeon, would come home from the hospital describing some of his surgical trainees as great, and some as frightening. Mark saw how disappointed his father was in the quality of some of his newest trainees, and was struck by society's acceptance and obliviousness to the disparity. For years, the fact that good and bad doctors alike would go forth and practice medicine with little oversight intrigued him. Mark later went to medical school, detouring to graduate school to study public health issues of quality control in medicine. He has won the respect of his peers in quality research and clinical practice throughout his career. He rose quickly through the ranks to become health commissioner of New York State.

As commissioner, Mark and his team wanted to address the horrific patterns of bad outcomes they had heard about in some of the state's heart hospitals. Doing heart bypass surgery was highly lucrative, and many hospitals were getting into the business when they probably shouldn't have. Concerned about the trend, doctors and nurses argued that the worst performing hospitals should have been referring heart-surgery patients to centers with dedicated teams and better outcomes. But patient outcomes had never been formally measured before. Like most state health departments, Chassin and his team received individual complaints about preventable deaths, but it was challenging to do anything about it given the big stakeholders in health care and their office's limited resources. Even if they had abundant resources, no one, including themselves, liked the idea of a government regulation aimed at micromanaging bad hospitals.

Mark didn't want to do the standard sluggish investigation of bad heart hospitals and slap wrists based on technicalities. He decided to do something radical—*make heart-surgery death rates public.*

Beginning in 1989, Mark and his team required all heart hospitals in the state to disclose their death rates from a heart operation known as coronary artery bypass graft procedure (CABG). Unlike other procedures where many variables are involved and for which the mortality statistic may unfairly purport to measure quality of care, an elective CABG is a highly standardized and commonly performed operation. Thus, for CABG procedures, a high death rate is closely associated with bad judgment, bad skill, and/or bad recovery care. It is a challenging operation with little room for error: If any one of a number of technical, medication, or electric-pacing mistakes occurs, the heart stops and the patient dies. But in the modern era of anesthesia and advanced surgical techniques, dying as a result of CABG *should* be a rare occurrence.

Mark's New York health commission also compiled hospital volumes—how many heart operations a hospital does each year, together with the complexity of its cases—and made the information available to the public. Death rates were mathematically adjusted for case complexity to make hospital comparisons fair. Now consumers could look up how many CABG operations a hospital did and what their risk-adjusted death rate was. The goal was to expose extreme outliers to consumers and let the free market work. And work it did indeed.

The first year that New York's hospitals were required to report heart-surgery death rates, wide variation was found—the death rate by hospital ranged from 1 percent to 18 percent—confirming long-standing rumors that quality of cardiac surgery was wildly variable among hospitals: Some places were outstanding while others were clearly flying by the seat of their pants. The high-mortality hospitals stood to lose millions of dollars in business. Consumers, armed with useful data, could now ask themselves this question: "Why have a CABG operation at a place where you have a one-in-six chance of dying compared to a hospital with a one-in-a-hundred chance of dying?"

Instantly, New York heart hospitals with high mortality rates scrambled to improve. Hospital executives held meetings with heart surgeons, nurses, and techs to try to find out what they had to do to improve care. Chassin's team offered support for poorly performing hospitals that were making the effort to improve by sending a team of heart-surgery experts to visit them. At one hospital, the staff reported that one surgeon's very high mortality rate was just because he wasn't fit to be operating. His mortality rate was so high, it was skewing the hospital's average overall. His hospital administrators ordered him, point-blank, to stop doing heart surgery.

The result of the release of this data? Big, broad improvements in mortality, statewide.[1] With each passing year of public reporting, the state's average death rate went down. In addition, bad outliers, like the hospital with the 18 percent mortality, were reined in.

The University of Rochester's Strong Memorial Hospital's mortality rate was worse than the state average. When administrators dug deeper, they discovered that two particular surgeons were skewing the rate. Neither doctor was trained in adult heart surgery—they were told to stop practicing adult heart operations. The hospital average improved overnight.

Winthrop-University Hospital was yet another embarrassed outlier in New York's public reporting program. When their 9 percent death rate hit the newspapers, the administration knew they needed to act fast. They hired their first full-time heart surgery chief from Yale, who revamped their program by setting up a team system for picking candidates for surgery. Before each operation, he personally reviewed the case with the patient's surgeon. Most important and despite the expense, hospital administrators gave the new surgery chief the dedicated heart nurses, heart anesthesiologists, and heart physician assistants he requested—a complete heart team. Mortality decreased from 9 percent to 2 percent. In short, on its own the hospital made all the changes it needed to get it right—in details that the state's health commission could never have anticipated, mandated, or enforced through regulation.

At St. Peter's Hospital, the elective-heart-surgery death rate met the state average, but emergency heart operations showed an alarming 26 percent death rate. On internal review, it was found that doctors weren't taking enough time to stabilize patients before surgery. Changes were made, and by the next year mortality for emergency cases dropped to zero.

Erie County Medical Center was the state's worst-performing hospital, with an overall 18 percent mortality rate—higher than that of soldiers wounded in the Iraq war. With its awful numbers now out in the open, on the Internet, the hospital's administrators acted swiftly to resuscitate its heart program. Hospital management listened to its frontline personnel, hired a new chief and some new dedicated staff, and instituted internal review conferences. Remarkably, within three years the mortality rate was cut to 7 percent, and in the years since, it has fallen to 1.7 percent.

New York's transparency program changed the way heart hospitals compete. No longer were they competing over highway billboards and valet parking. Suddenly they were competing over good outcomes. Resources were dedicated to fixing root problems, and bad heart-surgery centers cleaned up their acts. Hospitals started to do the hard work of assembling the clinical teams that doctors and nurses were asking for and promoting teamwork. They analyzed the mortality spreads among their surgeons and called doctors who were both way above and way below the average into meetings to discuss why. In a few cases, the worst outliers were removed. It worked. Introducing transparency to New York's heart centers brought something very novel and powerful to health care: public accountability.

Sustained Benefit in New York

Despite hospitals howling in protest when Chassin's program was announced, future patients benefited from the transparency. Statewide, deaths from heart surgery fell by 41 percent during the first four years of New York's public reporting program and have continued to decrease ever since.[2] In short, transparency made hospitals take a close look at their heart-surgery services. Poorly performing centers were forced to either clean house or shut down. Some public health researchers worried that closings would result in decreased access to heart surgery in rural areas. But as it turned out, many poor performers were in urban areas where there were other, better centers anyway. Some doctors learned how to game the system, and vocal critics cited this unintended consequence as the leading reason the public should not have access to the information. But as the program matured, loopholes and cheating were minimized.

Today, the nation's largest association of heart and lung surgeons (the Society of Thoracic Surgeons, or STS) collects reliable heart-surgery outcomes by hospital. They are impeccably accurate—and telling. Nearly every U.S. hospital that performs heart surgery participates in this proprietary registry. Individual hospital results are generated and returned to the hospital so they can compare their performance to national benchmarks—a process that now exists for many medical specialties. To make sure comparisons are fair, the surgeons' association also developed a way to mathematically account for a hospital's patient population, based on their disease complexity and risk, silencing the my-patients-are-sicker argument. The bottom line is that the STS national program to measure hospital outcomes is widely respected by doctors. But this valuable information is not available to the public unless you live in New York, or your local heart-surgery center participates in voluntary public reporting. Admirably, the STS has taken the bold stand to say on their website that the society "believes the public has a right to know the quality of surgical outcomes and considers public reporting an ethical responsibility of the specialty."[3] However, only one third of heart centers have voluntarily allowed their outcomes to be posted on the STS website, presumably the best centers. Despite the progress of the STS and other doctor groups, public reporting remains voluntary for hospitals.

Clearly, New York's early experiment had worked. Within a few years of boldly publishing hospital outcomes, New York had the lowest risk-adjusted mortality rate in the United States for CABG surgery. The free market forced quick and dramatic improvements—and the public won because patients finally were making informed decisions about where to go for their care. New York's transparency program for heart surgery represents the country's first experiment in public reporting in medicine.

Before New York's public reporting program, the science and method used to perform a CABG operation had not changed for years. What propelled better safety of the CABG operation wasn't new technology or new techniques. It was an even more radical innovation: public information. Forced to be accountable for their outcomes, hospitals were suddenly threatened with loss of business. Before then, they'd profited year after year, despite terrible outcomes, only because consumers walked in blind. Those days were now over. Embarrassed by high mortality rates, hospitals were forced to study their problems and figure out how to get things right. Hospital managers began talking to their heart surgeons. Everyone started to cooperate on improving outcomes. Administrators developed a previously unheard-of distaste for mediocrity, coupling crackdowns with unprecedented generosity in giving doctors and nurses their wish lists in resources and new ways of doing things that would let them do their job better.

Dr. Mark Chassin's social experiment in New York shows how simple accountability can transform a health care market. California and a few other states are now following New York's example, attempting to make the information user-friendly for consumers.[4]

To most doctors, Chassin is now a celebrated pioneer in this field. For his accomplishments, he was recently named CEO of the very prestigious and powerful organization the Joint Commission, the nation's hospital-accrediting body. But nationwide, transparency remains an uphill battle, mostly limited by the public's lack of knowledge that good metrics now exist.

Internal Crackdown

What motivates a CEO to leave his or her office and walk through a poorly performing "danger zone" of the hospital to ask frontline people what they need to deliver better care? One reason is public reporting.

If you want to see a hospital jump to enact large-scale reform, just watch when a journalist cracks open the story of bad medical care. In my years as a doctor, I've never seen hospital administrators move as fast as they do when their public image needs repair. It's the code blue for hospital administration. Yet it is rare. It takes a baby getting stolen from the newborn nursery, or an instrument left inside a patient showing up on an X-ray and later on CNN. In short, hospitals move fast when anything embarrassing or tragic gets into the public eye. During New York's transparency experiment, hospital CEOs started walking through the intensive care units asking the cardiac nurses why they had such high postsurgical mortality rates.

People are often surprised to learn this, but doctors and nurses crave administrative crackdowns. That's because they're moments of mutual communication that momentarily bridge the divide between workers and administrators and let them work together to fix problems. For hospital staff, it means someone will finally listen to them: about what they need on the ward, about making sure that whatever tragedy just occurred will never happen again, and about cracks in the system that concern them. When bosses with the clout to fire employees get involved in problem solving, things do get fixed. As a physician, I love it when an administrator comes to me and asks, "What can I do to make your department safer?" Sometimes the solutions are as simple as keeping the door to an operating room unlocked for emergencies, or assigning an extra nurse to an understaffed "danger zone" of the hospital. All it takes is some old-fashioned hands-on involvement.

The safety-culture survey used in the previously described Johns Hopkins safety study includes a few questions about the relationship between administration and hospital workers: for instance, "Is management responsive to your safety concerns?" The answer, we found, correlates to patient complication rates. Often, transparency just means using common sense—listening to your frontline workers.

Perceptions of Management

There is no greater champion of a good workplace culture in medicine than Dr. Bill Brody. During his tenure as president of the Johns Hopkins University, Dr. Brody rewarded hospital employees who acted on their patient-safety concerns.

One area of my hospital—the cardiac-surgery ICU—had serious problems. As measured by the survey, the cardiac ICU at Hopkins had poor safety-culture scores as measured by the employee survey. Nurse turnover was high, and complaints about patient care abounded. Infection rates were sky-high. Trainees hated working there. One told me it was his worst rotation in his five-year training program at Hopkins. Everyone at Hopkins seemed to know about it—even people who didn't work at Hopkins knew we had problems in the cardiac ICU. Staff in the unit had a high turnover rate, as if it was a sure road to burnout. It had an international reputation as one of the premier places to have heart surgery in the world, but hospital leadership became increasingly disturbed by the reality of poor safety-culture scores and proliferating stories of the medical mistakes that went on there.

Frustrated, Bill Brody got involved. Dr. Brody had a special fondness for cardiac surgery. Long before being named president, he had trained as a cardiac surgeon. Brody often waxes nostalgic about the old days of impeccable standards and strong teamwork in heart surgery, back in the days of the giants. Patient outcomes had indeed been superb under the direction of his mentors. When he returned to the cardiac ICU as president at Hopkins, he was blown away by how hazardous the care now was. "It was a disaster," he said. "No one was in charge. Nobody was really in charge of the patient." Reminiscing about his training days in cardiac surgery, he asked, "How did we get to be so bad?"[5]

Determined to fix the problem, and despite his eminent position as president of the mammoth institution, Brody got out from behind his desk and walked over to the unit. He began rounding through the cardiac-surgery unit every week. He met with staff and talked with them about safety concerns, the occurrence of medical errors, and the high infection rate. On one of these days, he saw that lights in one of the operating rooms were dirty.

"I can't get housekeeping to take care of it," one nurse told him, adding hopefully, "Can *you* call housekeeping to take care of it?"

The episode told Dr. Brody that people in the unit needed to feel that they had the right to call a time-out and stop a procedure from starting whenever they had a safety concern—the same way Toyota factory workers are empowered to stop the assembly line if they have a safety concern. Shocked that hospital workers would knowingly let patients enter a dirty operating room—a sure route to potentially life-threatening infections—Dr. Brody instructed them to cancel surgery whenever any one of them believed it was unsafe to proceed. As soon as the nurse notified him, someone came to replace the dirty bulb, cleaned up, and the case proceeded.

The problem, he found, was just that no one felt comfortable speaking up. Nurses complained that the equipment was antiquated, the rooms were small, and the trainees were in over their heads. Yet staff didn't feel they had the right to do anything about these matters for themselves. Until Dr. Brody spent many days in the unit with them, they all felt management was unresponsive to their concerns. After Brody, as a top official, came on the ward to directly communicate his desire to back them up, they

began to feel empowered to act on their concerns, either themselves directly or by complaining to management.

Dr. Brody listened to people and also put himself to work. It
was a radical step to get the unit back on track. He continued to
spend one day a week at the unit, making sure the correct equipment was ordered, that employees were better able to do their jobs
safely, and that the trainees felt supported in their workloads. Dr.
Brody kept this up until the culture scores improved and infection rates declined. Because of his willingness to leave his fancy
office and engage with frontline workers, Hopkins once again
became a high-quality hospital to have cardiac surgery.

After Dr. Brody was reasonably satisfied with the improvements in the unit, my research partner, safety advocate Dr. Peter
Pronovost, was named director of the unit. Today care is better,
patients are safer, and doctors and nurses have what they need to
do their jobs—all because of a successful internal crackdown and
a model leader who wasn't afraid to roll up his sleeves and respond to his staff's concerns.

Like Gulf Coast oil-spill cleanups, such hospital crackdowns are
rarely altruistic. They are commonly triggered by fears of a tarnished public image. When rumor had it that Medicare was going
to make hospital infection rates public, American hospital administrators jumped. The leading cause of infection is a failure of
health care workers simply to wash their hands. Prevention is easy,
so long as you are vigilant about hand washing. It's nineteenth-
century, not twenty-first-century, science—but it works.

After the rumor of infection rates going public was confirmed
for a few select types of surgery, I couldn't help but notice administrators suddenly doing much more walking on the units, asking
nurses and doctors what it would take to get everyone to wash
their hands and reduce the infection rate. Within a week, alcohol
and sterilizing-lotion hand-washing dispensers appeared at every
corner of the hospital—425 of them. Posters were put up everywhere espousing the benefits of clean hands. Every computer
screen saver was programmed with the motto REMEMBER TO WASH
YOUR HANDS.

The internal crackdown I witnessed worked. Infection rates

were cut in half at my hospital and at many others. *But infections are just one of dozens of commonly preventable bad patient outcomes,* all of which should be made public knowledge. With universal transparency, hospital leadership would also develop a fast-moving protocol by which to conduct crackdowns whenever new problems come to light. Sunlight, it is often said, is the best disinfectant. But under our current, largely unaccountable system, hospital problems out of sight and out of mind just pile up until they get so out of hand, only a major, punishing scandal can hope to remedy them.

Walter Reed

Walter Reed Army Medical Center was famous as the leading hospital for our nation's military personnel. Every wartime president of the United States takes a highly publicized tour of Walter Reed. The hospital treated ailing and wounded servicemen and women, most in their twenties and thirties, the prime of their lives, dealing with some of the most painful and life-changing injuries possible to body and mind. Most Americans believed that Walter Reed was top-notch, delivering the utmost in quality care to their nation's war heroes. But that's not what they would have heard from Walter Reed nurses working in Building 18.

As a surgical resident at a neighboring hospital in the early 2000s, I knew the employees in Walter Reed's outpatient areas felt their hospital's safety culture was atrocious. Jessica, a nurse, told me of her concern about the gross neglect of soldiers there—it was sickening to hear about blind amputees with severe psychiatric conditions being given complicated instructions about finding multiple offices just to get essential medication. The more nurses, techs, and other health professionals I met from Walter Reed, the more stories I heard about some of the rooms veterans lived in at the medical center—horror stories of medical neglect, substandard care, and patients falling through the cracks. Building 18, in particular, was known to be the worst "danger zone" at the medical center. Accounts of what was happening there were heart-wrenching, and every employee had a tale to tell. Dr. Michael Marohn, a colleague of mine at Johns Hopkins, had worked at Walter Reed and told me how he had voiced concerns about the appalling patient care in Building 18, but to his dismay, nothing there got better.

A 2005 story on *Salon* hinted that there was a serious problem when First Lieutenant Julian Goodrum was interviewed about his court martial for seeking medical care elsewhere due to Walter Reed's abysmal conditions.[6] Then in 2007, the *Washington Post* grabbed the nation's attention when it exposed Walter Reed's problems in detail in a blistering series of investigative pieces. While nonmedical friends I knew said, "I can't believe it," I thought, Many of us have known about this for years.

SOLDIERS FACE NEGLECT, FRUSTRATION AT ARMY'S TOP MEDICAL FACILITY was the *Post*'s headline on its first story. Mold, insects, and dilapidated conditions were exposed in this important article. Accounts of patients ignored or forgotten. The networks covered it as a top story for days. It was a national disgrace. President George W. Bush addressed the nation about it. The secretary of the army was fired and the secretary of defense was rumored to be next. The scandal shook the country. Americans finally learned what Walter Reed nurses and other staff had known for many years: Walter Reed Hospital Building 18 was a very dangerous place.

Creating Systemic Change

If Walter Reed employees had taken the safety-culture survey—available, ironically, on one of the government's own websites—and the results had been made public, everyone would have known about its problems years before any excoriating exposé needed to break. Walter Reed would have been made accountable before things got as bad as they did. How many people might have been saved from terrible treatment? Thankfully, the public outcry after the Walter Reed exposé did force it to clean up its act. But most bad hospitals don't suffer newspaper publicity like Walter

Reed's. In fact, from what I've seen since my internship, little has changed at the "chop shops" and other "danger zones" I once rotated through as a resident in training. Lacking accountability— and thus the discipline of the market—these hospitals continue to conduct business as usual that is substandard.

CHAPTER 4

The Supersurgeon and the Shah

IF EVER THERE WERE A SUPERDOCTOR in medicine, it was famed Texas surgeon Michael DeBakey. He died in 2008 at the age of ninety-nine. As head of the surgical department at his Texas hospital, he performed a record total of fifty thousand operations in his life. He was the twentieth century's most celebrated pioneer of a number of surgical procedures, operating-room instruments, and medical devices. Like most surgeons, almost every day I ask my nurse for a "DeBakey" and am handed a DeBakey forceps— one of my favorite instruments. Nearly every surgeon in the world uses it, a brilliantly designed surgical forceps and a staple of every operating-room instrument tray.

Considered by many to be the greatest surgeon in the world, Dr. DeBakey had been summoned to operate on Soviet leader Boris Yeltsin and many other famous heads of state. Worldwide, patients in need of surgery would beg and plead to have Dr. De-Bakey perform their operations. Hollywood celebrities and politicians pulled every string to get to him.

In 1969, Dr. DeBakey was awarded the Presidential Medal of Freedom, and in 2007 he was recognized with the Congressional Gold Medal for his contributions to science and medicine. These two distinctions are considered to be the highest civilian awards in the United States.

In 1978, His Majesty Mohammad Reza Pahlavi, the Shah of Iran, was considered one of the most important figures in the

world to the U.S. government. He was an attractive man who
wore distinguished suits and dined with the world's elite. Besides
controlling a valuable spigot of oil that fueled the U.S. economy,
the Shah was a critical U.S. ally in the Cold War and the pivotal
figure in the balance of power in the Middle East. In fact, the CIA
had gone to the lengths of covertly implementing a coup d'état in
1953 to topple the Mossadeq regime and install the Shah on the
throne. Since then, the U.S. and its key allies had relied on His
Majesty to control political elements unfriendly to the U.S. and
to advance Washington's interests in the region. With massive
American support, the Shah ruled for thirty-three years.

When the Shah suddenly fell ill, Washington faced a potential
international crisis. Pahlavi was admitted to a fourteen-suite VIP
floor at a well-known Middle Eastern hospital. The U.S. acted swiftly
to ensure that he got the best care. A medical team including David
Rockefeller's private doctor and DeBakey sped to the Middle East
in a chartered Boeing 707 jet to pick up the Shah. The key world
figure and the world-famous surgeon seemed well matched.

Upon seeing the Shah, Dr. DeBakey recommended immediate
surgery to remove his spleen. The main pitfall of any spleen operation is the possibility that the surgeon could inadvertently
cut the tail of the pancreas, which lies in direct proximity to the
spleen. This can lead to a fatal infection weeks later from the pancreas slowly leaking pancreatic fluid. Standard good practice has
long called for the surgeon to place a surgical drain in the area of
the pancreas to prevent pancreatic fluid from accumulating in
case it is inadvertently cut.[1]

Dr. DeBakey did not take this simple, standard safety measure.
Even though the Shah's spleen was exceptionally large, increas-
ing the risk of a pancreas injury, DeBakey refused to leave a
drain, as he was confident he would never touch the pancreas.
After the one-hour-and-twenty-minute operation, he reported that
it went "about as smoothly as you could make it" and that the
Shah "couldn't be better."[2] Dr. DeBakey was an instant hero to
Middle Easterners and a savior of U.S. diplomatic relations.

For his successful operation, Dr. DeBakey received a heralded
medal of honor from the president of Egypt, the highest honor for

a civilian. Soon after DeBakey received these kudos, however, the Shah began to experience fevers and vomiting. Then he got worse. His local Egyptian doctors sampled the fluid that had built up in the area of the operation and determined that it came from a leaking pancreas. The fluid had accumulated and as a result became infected. The French doctors caring for the ailing Shah criticized Dr. DeBakey for not placing the standard surgical drain at the time of the operation—a simple thing to do that would have prevented his deterioration from the festering, now infected, fluid. The Shah's family, now distrustful of the care provided by the Americans, called a French team of doctors to care for His Majesty. The French doctors agreed with the local Egyptian doctors that Dr. DeBakey had accidentally cut the pancreas and should have placed a surgical drain to prevent the complication.

Under pressure from Egypt and the United States, Dr. DeBakey returned to see his now deteriorating patient. The Shah had lost a lot of weight and looked terrible. An Islamic revolution back in Iran was taking advantage of the Shah's apparent illness, evident to anyone who saw his appearance. But Dr. DeBakey refused to believe that the Shah had a pancreatic fluid leak, telling the Shah's family that his malaise was likely due to toxicity from medication the Shah was receiving against DeBakey's recommendation. The Shah's health worsened from the infected fluid until he was completely debilitated.

Doctors from all over the world now became involved, many critical of DeBakey. The international medical imbroglio over what went wrong during DeBakey's surgery and how to handle it was complicated by a growing American frustration over the hostages in Iran. In the Shah's home country, the rising Ayatollah Khomeini criticized the Shah's doctors and the country of Egypt for hosting his care, calling those who helped him satanic. Washington worried that more public criticism of the American care of the Shah could jeopardize the safety of the American hostages.

After a three-month delay in diagnosis littered with controversy, a French surgeon reopened the Shah's wound and let out 1.5 liters of pus and infected pancreatic tissue. It was clear that Dr. DeBakey had inadvertently cut the pancreas during his operation.

But by this point it was also too late, and the infection—combined with the Shah's worsening lymphoma—had taken a heavy toll on him. He died weeks later, an event that sparked an international episode over what went wrong, adding to the turmoil in U.S. foreign policy.

What the Shah and the State Department failed to realize was that Dr. DeBakey was a cardiovascular surgeon, *not* an abdominal surgeon. His greatness stemmed from his innovation in heart and vascular surgery, not in spleen or pancreas surgery. In fact, compared to surgeons who specialized in the abdomen, Dr. DeBakey had little experience operating on the spleen, even less experience operating on a cancerous spleen, and almost no experience operating on the pancreas.

In researching his many contributions to medicine, I discovered that, out of the record-breaking 479 articles DeBakey wrote, more than 95 percent were about cardiovascular surgery. Only one was about the spleen (and he was not one of the lead authors). Dr. DeBakey should have referred the Shah to a surgeon who did a lot of spleen removals. Alternatively, the Shah or his family should have insisted on a doctor who did a lot of spleen removals. Instead, even the most powerful heads of state were dazzled by the allure of the superstar surgeon, placing adoration of a celebrity and assumptions about his brand over common sense.

A recent landmark research study published in the *New England Journal of Medicine* solidified what most doctors and nurses already knew. Using national data, a leading health-services research group from the University of Michigan found that surgical death rates are directly related to a surgeon's experience with that particular operation. The researchers compared death rates after an operation against the surgeon's experience with that specific operation.

The researchers found the same relationship for many types of surgical procedures. The rarer the condition, the more experience mattered. Indeed, "practice makes perfect" is a golden rule for medical procedures. In fact, one of the secondary findings of New York State's public reporting experiment in heart surgery was that high-volume doctors performed much better than low-volume

Death Rate after Pancreas Surgery
by Surgeon Experience

	Death Rate
Surgeons who perform fewer than two operations per year	14.7 percent
Surgeons who perform two to four operations per year	8.5 percent
Surgeons who perform more than four operations per year	4.6 percent

Source: John D. Birkmeyer et al., "Surgeon Volume and Operative Mortality in the United States," *New England Journal of Medicine* 349, no. 22 (2003) 2117–27.

doctors. In fact, Dr. Mark Chassin's program observed that low-volume heart surgeons recorded a mortality rate four times higher than the state average.[3]

But doesn't volume transparency hurt new doctors fresh out of training? my students have sometimes asked me. The model partially being restored in American medicine today is for new doctors (fully certified to work independently) to pair up with more experienced doctors to get a bit of "volume" under their belts before doing procedures alone. Thus a paired team of doctors imparts the "volume" experience to both the less experienced and the more experienced doctor. I admire young doctors who do this. Having learned the wrong way myself—from the trial and error of *practicing on live patients alone as an intern*—I am a firm believer that there are equally effective ways to educate doctors that don't use patients as guinea pigs. The apprenticeship approach has not only been the way doctors have trained for centuries, but it is also established practice in Asia, Europe, and elsewhere. There, surgeons complete their official training and will often pair up with senior surgeons to do complex procedures before doing them on their own. This more humble (albeit less profitable) approach improves safety. It also contrasts the prevailing American training motto every doctor knows: "See one, do one, teach one."

Many of my more experienced colleagues agree, it is better to learn from the wisdom of others than by making mistakes practicing on patients. Training wheels work. Moreover, similar to advanced cockpit simulators that train pilots, new state-of-the-art patient simulators work beautifully for medical training. But sadly, only a few teaching hospitals use them, mostly for reasons of—you guessed it—cost.

Volume matters. As a homeowner, you wouldn't hire a plumber to fix your fuse box. The plumber's error could easily cause a spark that could burn your house to the ground. Yet every day there are patients sitting in waiting rooms waiting for the wrong doctor to treat their condition. And every day, patients sit in waiting rooms at the wrong hospital for what they need done. Yet the uninformed public has little choice.

Volume also matters in all medical care, not just procedures. When seeking care for a possible stroke, persistent cough, or possible tick bite, you should be able to look on the national Hospital Compare website (www.hospitalcompare.hhs.gov) to see how many cases of stroke, pneumonia, or Lyme disease each medical center in your area treats each year. But currently you can't because hospitals don't disclose that information. Say your mother develops a stroke. If you see that hospital A sees six cases per year and hospital B treats one hundred cases of stroke per year, you know where to go. Or imagine you got a tick bite and a hospital one hour away saw twenty-five cases last year, whereas a closer hospital saw zero cases last year. Trust me, that volume differential matters, especially for major conditions. The differences in the care you receive can be shocking.

Even the most reputable hospital may have at least one or two departments in shambles and struggling for survival. Such departments rely on the weight of the overall institution to keep patients coming in the door. If a struggling department does finally die, the hospital operator will politely say they no longer offer that service, or that it is being offered through a "partnership" with a private-practice group in the community. One "cancer center" that I know of hung on based on just one low-volume, grumpy oncologist who finally decided to quit.

While volume never tells the whole story, it can be used in combination with other metrics such as hospital employee-safety attitudes, hospital complication rates, and hospital readmission rates. There is no compelling reason why all of this data can't be posted online for everyone to see.

CHAPTER 5

"How I Like to Do It"

Gretchen and Ronald

EVERY DAY IN AMERICA, PEOPLE LAND in doctors' offices by pure happenstance and get widely divergent recommendations, depending on who is doing the exam. If you have a sore knee, Doctor A may tell you to "try to stay off it" while Doctor B may suggest a knee surgery. This nonstandardized approach to treatment sometimes reflects medical art, but in other cases, one person is getting good care and the other isn't.

Ever since I've been in medicine, I've been amazed that each doctor has their own personal threshold to give a blood transfusion to patients with anemia, or low blood level, despite established guidelines. Many surgeons have hard-and-fast rules: "I like to transfuse everyone with a blood level below seven" or "I like to transfuse everyone with a blood level below twelve"—rules I have heard and continue to hear frequently. Based on evidence in the *New England Journal of Medicine* outlining specific criteria, most hospitals are overusing their blood supply. Americans are continually urged to donate blood to "save lives," but the so-called national blood shortage crisis may really be more of a national blood overuse crisis.

The surgeon and researcher Dr. Atul Gawande of Harvard perfectly demonstrated the stark differences in medical judgment in a 2009 study of two cities in Texas. Both cities were comparable in their populations, socioeconomic status, and health outcomes. What was striking was that these two practically identical towns had radically different numbers of medical procedures and health care costs. One town, McAllen, was racking up almost double the costs of its twin, El Paso.[1] Critics worked hard to see if one town was less healthy than the other, or if the discrepancy could perhaps be blamed on a cluster of bad-apple docs. No matter the angle from which the data was reviewed, the conclusion remained the same—the towns were roughly equivalent. The only reason for massive expenditures in one city and relative economy in the other was that some doctors just do more stuff, and so do entire *hospitals*.

I took in this painful lesson while on rotation at a university-affiliated community hospital where I met Gretchen, a sweet young woman who needed breast-cancer surgery. Gretchen had absolute faith that she was receiving care in a top-quality medical center. When I asked her why she chose this particular hospital for her procedure, she explained that the hospital's home page displayed the logo of its prestigious affiliate university saying its center had a number-one ranking. My ears perking up over a "ranking," I pressed her further about it, but its source sounded nebulous to me. When I got back to the office to look it up, I found that this hospital's administration had simply undertaken a public relations campaign to market itself as having a "comprehensive breast cancer center." This had led to an essentially bogus ranking pasted on the home page of its website, apparently out of a medical-services-oriented web designer's form kit.

What? "Comprehensive"? "Center"? I was shocked at the fancy branding, since I worked there and knew it was little better equipped than a school nurse's office. The facility did not have a National Cancer Institute designation as a cancer center, only the faux marketing claims of one by calling its skeleton breast-cancer staff a "center."

I was bothered by the disingenuous nature of the hospital's marketing—and worried for Gretchen. I gently asked her if she considered going to some other cancer centers, but I knew in doing so I was walking on thin ice with my own job.

Nothing at this "comprehensive cancer center" was coordinated, established, or noteworthy. It takes an army of dedicated radiologists, oncologists, breast surgeons, and genetic counselors to create a true state-of-the-art comprehensive breast-cancer center—this hospital did only a few dozen breast operations a year. True centers perform hundreds of procedures to get recognition as a center of excellence. They should, for instance, be ahead of the curve in utilization of effective new technology. They should offer participation in national clinical trials, along with state-of-the-art plastic surgery to reconstruct the breast in a way that feels and looks right.

As Gretchen prepared for her breast-removal procedure, I couldn't help but see that this hospital didn't even have the equipment to perform any of the newer, minimally invasive techniques such as the stereotactic biopsy. Even more worrisome, the plastic surgeons at this institution didn't know how to do an advanced breast-reconstruction procedure called the DIEP flap (deep inferior epigastric perforators flap)—an operation with well-established, superior outcomes commonly performed in about half of U.S. cancer centers. The DIEP flap uses the body's natural tissue and blood supply, using small blood vessels in the abdomen, to re-create a breast. It results in the best feel, contour, cosmetics, and long-term function of any breast-reconstruction operation available now. I would highly recommend breast reconstruction with a DIEP flap if my mother or a dear friend had to have a breast removed. This reconstructive operation requires a highly trained plastic surgeon. To perform the DIEP-flap procedure usually requires a year of subspecialty training above and beyond plastic surgery training. The procedure also requires an expensive surgical microscope to reconnect the small blood vessels.

Gretchen's hospital didn't own the microscope, and her charming plastic surgeons didn't know how to do the DIEP flap. Not only did they not have the in-house expertise to give her the surgery she needed and deserved, they didn't bother to tell her that she could have had this superior treatment at another hospital several miles away. Doctors at the neighboring hospital had both the microscope and the surgeons to do her surgery with the best result. The breast specialists there did more than three hundred breast operations a year using the superior DIEP-flap reconstruction procedure, and their outcomes reflected it. The nearby hospital also offered all the latest chemotherapy clinical trials.

Gretchen wound up at a bad hospital for her condition, one whose culture prioritized keeping patients' business over delivering the best care. If she had simply known the right information to be an educated consumer of medicine, Gretchen could have gotten in her car and driven those few miles to a better outcome. Instead she stayed where she was, and her reconstructed breast came out looking permanently unnatural. When I asked her if she was pleased with the result, she said, "I don't really know what to compare it to, but yes, I feel very blessed."

Gretchen's story taught me a personal lesson. When choosing a hospital, beware of clever marketing. When a company wants to sell soda or a designer wants to market its two-hundred-dollar blue jeans, they will pump endless amounts of money into advertising campaigns to make their product appealing to consumers. Hospitals are no different but, unlike choosing a pair of jeans, choosing the wrong health care provider can have permanent consequences. Don't be taken in by fancy banners like "center," "top hospital," or "best docs." Insist on finding out how many patients they treat each year for your condition. Hospitals create "centers" to lure business, but remember, one doctor—or even a few—does not constitute a "comprehensive center." Patient-satisfaction surveys do not capture quality medical care, and "top" scores and rankings in magazines are often paid for.

Not for the first time in my career, I felt the weight of ethics on my shoulders like an incubus. I desperately wanted to tell Gretchen to go elsewhere. But I did not. I knew that referring her elsewhere would violate the resident's code of omertà and get me in big trouble, maybe even fired. I was an unknown employee to the hospital. Telling her to go elsewhere would have made me very well-known by superiors evaluating me, my teachers, and the hospital management—and a marked man. It would be akin to a Ford salesman telling an eager buyer who shows up in the salesroom to go buy a Honda, except that Gretchen's medical care had a much larger profit margin at stake for the hospital than a new-car sale would have for a dealership.

In too many areas of our medical culture, the combination of pride and perverse incentives against referring patients to the best place for care is strong. While a few hospitals are now moving to a fixed-salary system for their doctors, the failure to refer patients to a more suitable facility is still rampant in medicine. As I rotated through more departments such as plastics, orthopedics, neurosurgery, ear-nose-and-throat, and urology (about fifty rotations in all), and five more hospitals, it became clear to me that under-referring was the rule, not the exception. Sure, referring went on all the time, but to doctors in other fields of medicine.

I had seen this failure to refer in other professions before, such as when a lawyer took on my friend's divorce case without telling him that he'd never been involved in a divorce case before (corporate litigation was his specialty). On a personal level, I remember meeting a real estate agent who wouldn't concede she didn't know anything about the neighborhood in which I wanted to buy. Luckily, I was able to see through her claims and switched to another agent who had sold dozens of homes in that area. Clearly, the first agent didn't want to let on her lack of knowledge so as to not lose my business—a common less-than-honest practice. I had always thought medicine was a noble exception to the pride and greed of under-referring, but I was wrong. Over time, I learned that suboptimal care—even when better care was known to be just a referral away—was ubiquitous.

When I try to forgive myself for failing Gretchen, I like to think I had good reasons at the time: I'd heard of what happened when someone before me took the high road. A trainee had encouraged a patient to go to another hospital for treatment and, like a delinquent student, had been sent to the chief's office to receive "couch time"—a dressing-down followed by being treated like a dunce and a pariah on his return to rotation. It is a harsh punishment in a field in which one's reputation with one's peers is everything. So I learned to swallow the bitter pill of accepting a hospital's shortcomings so as not to jeopardize my ability to advance in my career. I choked on that pill once again when, one evening in the emergency room, I met Ronald.

To fully understand Ronald's experience, one must understand what it's like to be on call for the emergency room. The standard 120-hour workweek transforms the most idealistic resident into a weary foot soldier struggling for survival, with mottos like "Get 'er done" and "Make it happen." The insistent buzzing of the ER pager puts you in a constant state of anxiety: Does that buzz mean it's time to be a hero? Or is it the opening knell of a nightmare situation? Perpetually exhausted, we had little time to question what we did—our lives revolved around the purely robotic execution of senior attending surgeons' orders, the ultimate reward for which was to have a higher-ranked surgeon tell us we were "strong."

I met Ronald in the ER one evening. He was a pleasant thirty-two-year-old athletic man who seemed completely healthy but for a protrusion at his belly button about the size of a grapefruit. "Chip shot," I told my friend who was the ER resident working with me. I'd seen it several times before. It's a common long-term complication in as many as 20 percent of all patients after abdominal surgery. Fortunately, there is an easy, minimally invasive fix, and I felt confident that Ronald would have a quick surgery and go home the same night.

I filled out an evaluation note on Ronald's chart using a pre-printed form, leaving the box entitled "plan" blank, as we usually did before we talked to the covering attending surgeon on call. Checking the night's schedule, I was glad to see that Dr. Kai was on call, a young surgeon with great outcomes who was very slick. "Slick" is our jargon for doing operations like these through a few small keyhole incisions using a small camera (a laparoscope) and long instruments. I was happy for Ronald to land Dr. Kai that night. We doctors can develop accelerated close relationships with our patients in the emergency room over problems like these, and this was one of those rewarding moments in the making. I got ready to comfort Ronald by explaining to him that Dr. Kai would do a minimally invasive operation within a few hours, and he'd probably be able to walk home the same day with a couple of Band-

Aids over his incisions. Then my coresident suddenly hooked me aside and delivered news that made my blood run cold.

"Shrek is on call tonight," he told me.

"What?" I exclaimed out loud before I could stop myself.

I'd read the schedule wrong. Dr. Kai had been on call the previous night. Instead, Ronald would be delivered to the hands of the doctor we called Shrek (nicknamed for his folded brow, cloddish appearance, and incomprehensible grunts). Shrek was about as knowledgeable in minimally invasive surgery as his cartoon namesake. Instead, he liked to do all operations through the big, open approach. His MO was to cut an incision the length of the whole abdomen, leaving two surgical drains in for weeks afterward. Instead of walking home the same day of a slick keyhole procedure by Dr. Kai, Ronald would now be in the hospital for a week to recover from Shrek's large incision.

As I cared for Ronald in recovery, I again felt the weight of my junior status when it came to being honest with him about his care. Ronald was in a lot of pain that week. In addition to the unnecessarily invasive quality of the open procedure he'd endured, the open operation also carried a higher risk that the entire abdominal closure could break down from a wound infection. On day three of his recovery, that is exactly what happened.

Infection is a dreaded complication requiring months of wound care, sometimes requiring reoperation. It is also totally preventable. The minimally invasive version of the procedure never results in an infection—the incisions are too small to allow it.

As I changed the open wound that spanned Ronald from stem to stern, I peeled off the gauze from the beefy, red wound, cringing a little at his clearly excruciating pain. It seemed so wrong. I felt frustrated, demoralized, and completely powerless. What could I do? Report Shrek to the chief of surgery? Call the president of the hospital? Plant a sign in front of the hospital, BEWARE OF SHREK?

I knew saying anything to our chief was political suicide, and that calling the hospital president was a stunt that would haunt my career. Washington's surgical community was small; if I was labeled as a whistle-blower, my career would be shot. I had witnessed other faculty complaining about the way Shrek operated, but their complaining fell on deaf ears (ears content with the high revenue Shrek brought in for the hospital). If senior faculty got nowhere with Shrek, how could I put a stop to his needlessly large operations? Exhausted by it all, I decided to look away and just do my job. I was being indoctrinated into the secretive culture of modern medicine.

In the end, Ronald endured a monthlong recovery marked by extraordinary pain, complications, inactivity, and lost time at work. I knew the hospital tracked wound-infection rates internally, but these rates were unknown to the public. If they had been known, people would have seen that Shrek's rate was around 20 percent, while Dr. Kai's—and every other surgeon who did the minimally invasive procedure—had a rate close to zero. "Ron," as he insisted I call him, would never know that if only he had come to the hospital on a different night of the week, he would have had a completely different operation and his recovery would have been radically different. But how *could* he know about the different "styles" of practicing medicine?

Ronald, like millions of Americans, might have avoided the nightmare he experienced if he had known exactly the right questions to ask:

- Are there other ways of treating this?
- What percent of these operations are done open versus the minimally invasive way in the U.S.?
- What percent of these operations do *you* do open versus the minimally invasive way?
- What are the differences in complication rates for each?
- How many days will I be in the hospital if I have it done one way versus the other?
- Can I get a second opinion while I'm here in the hospital?

The doctors who operated on Gretchen and Ronald angered me. I was bothered by the fact that they didn't just refer them to someone who could have done a safer and better operation. To let off steam, I shared my frustration over a drink with my fellow resident

Dr. Chris Benjamin. "Just keep your head down, Mart," he said. "We're not going to be helping anyone if we get kicked out of the residency program." He reminded me that we were making $29,000 a year in salary and had school debts. "We could be on the streets tomorrow. It's a messed-up, phony system and we're not going to change it," he said in his straight-talking Louisiana drawl.

So many times during my residency I wanted to tell patients to run away. Caring for the victims of unnecessary, sometimes entirely wrong, surgery wore me down. I took my medical-school graduation oath to "do no harm" seriously, so I was internally ashamed at how far I'd come from the days of telling my medical-school interviewer that I wanted to be a medical missionary. Ronald and Gretchen demonstrated to me the irony of "Do no harm"—it was a virtue at graduation, but a farce in the emergency room.

The 120-plus-hour workweek was grueling. "Survive" became our motto. But by the end of my training, I was rested, bolder, and more confident. I realized that medicine's culture was turning me into the doctor I didn't want to be, and I wasn't willing to sully the oath I took when I graduated from school. I made a pact with myself to just tell the patients who were on Gretchen's or Ronald's path, when appropriate, to take their things, walk out of the ER without checking out, and drive over to X hospital and to ask for Dr. Y.

Medicine's Garden of Eden

Jenn is an active young businesswoman I operated on two years ago for a pancreas mass called a neuroendocrine tumor. She had a wonderful experience with the surgery. As a result, she loves me and has been praising me on her Facebook page and Tweeting about how I was the answer to her prayers.

Recently, she came back to see me because she wasn't feeling well. I discovered she had since developed a liver tumor requiring more surgery. She begged me to do it. But it was a liver tumor in a slightly difficult location, and I tend only to tackle liver tumors when they are in an easy position, since I don't do much liver surgery anymore. (I'm rusty on my advanced liver surgery.) It could likely have been removed more safely by a surgeon who does more of that type of operation, not by me. My referral of her to a liver specialist would likely have decreased her complication risk from, say, 3 percent in my hands to 1 percent in his hands, but mean $3,000 less in income for me. Keep in mind that I, like all surgeons, am also statistically more likely to be overconfident about my skills than underconfident. This is a part of our DNA as surgeons. (As we say, we're always confident and usually right.)

I could have taken Jenn to surgery. It was tempting. I could have justified it ethically, because my success rate was still high. Malpractice risk was not a concern because my credentials and the consent forms she would sign would keep me bulletproof if a complication developed. Like all those patients who lined up for Hodad, she probably would have been grateful to me for doing her operation, no matter what happened. Certainly no one in my world would have had a problem with it if I had done the operation—no one ever reviewed my cases. It is a powerful vortex of temptation for a doctor: the appeal of doing what you love (operating), earning money ($3,000), and helping a grateful patient who is already begging you to do her surgery. See how hard it is?

I did refer Jenn to a liver surgeon, but these decisions are not as cut-and-dried as the economists and politicians would have you believe. While most doctors are good people, powerful financial and other incentives pull at us. The temptation to not refer is stronger now than ever—given declining doctor pay, a bankrupt Medicare and Medicaid system, higher malpractice premiums, medical-school debts, and escalating office costs.

If financial incentives were realigned so that revenue for Jenn's operation was distributed evenly to a group of doctors, I would guess the temptation not to refer would be greatly reduced. The idea of appropriate referrals recalls the scene in the classic holiday film *Miracle on 34th Street* when retail rivals Macy's and Gimbel's put aside their competition and chose to refer shoppers to each other if one didn't have the gift shoppers needed in stock. The result in the movie was that thankful shoppers patronized *both* stores with more devotion than before.

We doctors by nature are highly competitive individuals. After all, we outperformed droves of students to get to where we are. We ought to be competing over the quality and value of our services. What's best for patients is teamwork among doctors. Strangely, many hospitals try to disincentivize teamwork, since the sum of individual high productivity is a larger hospitalwide profit. I've occasionally suggested to hospitals that team conferences be added so that select recommendations to patients are reviewed by doctors as a group. This suggestion generally doesn't fly. The ideal model is seen today in multidisciplinary, multispecialty breast clinics, where one can see a range of breast doctors on the same visit. At Johns Hopkins, I have used the same thinking in connection with other medical conditions. Today multidisciplinary clinics, like the one I cofounded in my own specialty, are springing up around the country.

Fred Flintstone Care

When I ask friends how they choose a doctor, some say they go with the doctor with the most experience (as if they have read the *New England Journal of Medicine* studies I cite earlier). Choosing an experienced doctor certainly makes good sense. Yet there's one serious pitfall to choosing a doctor based purely on experience: Fred Flintstone care.

Fred Flintstone care is doctor speak for antiquated, outdated medicine. It's what one well-known political figure recently got when she underwent a major open operation to remove a small abdominal tumor. That small tumor could have been removed with a minimally invasive method with lower risks than a large open operation. But the chief of surgery emeritus had never learned how to do minimally invasive surgery.

Many surgeons I know don't offer patients minimally invasive or cutting-edge options only because they don't know how to do them. Further, the pattern of which doctors offer it and which doctors don't has no correlation with the prestige or size of the hospital in which they practice.

Fred Flintstone care is what one famous actress got when her aneurysm ruptured and the surgeon on call only knew how to do a big operation to cut her open and repair it. He had never learned how to fix such aneurysms through a wire and expandable stent through a leg vessel—a less invasive approach with fewer complications.

Fred Flintstone care is also what one patient got when I was in training and her doctor recommended that her gallbladder be removed through a large incision. When asked later at a weekly meeting in front of his peers why he didn't do it with a scope through a small keyhole incision, he shrugged and replied, "It's not as much fun." The room of surgeons broke out in a thunderous laugh.

Fred Flintstone care is what my friend Alex Fillmore received when he got appendicitis and underwent an open operation instead of a laparoscopic removal of the appendix. The surgeon on call that day told me he didn't believe the studies that showed laparoscopic procedures to be superior—even though, when I brought them up, he didn't know the studies existed.

As Ronald's experience with Shrek in the ER proved, Fred Flintstone care is more dangerous care and is more common among older, experienced surgeons who have routinized a procedure that, in the interim, may have been updated. To ensure you are not getting Fred Flintstone care, run a senior doctor's recommendation by a younger doctor to get validation and maybe learn about other, newer options.

We need transparency so that, for a given hospital and procedure, you can look up how many that hospital does and what percent are done minimally invasive compared to other hospitals and the national average. Until then, we are all forced to conduct amateur private investigations every time we need care. Google your medical condition to learn about a minimally invasive operation equivalent, then ask your doctor about it. If the doctor says he or she doesn't know how to do it—or doesn't believe in it—get a second opinion from someone who does do the procedure. All surgery has risks, so your goal should be to err on the side of less is more, unless the need for the more invasive procedure is very clear. Many procedures in medicine now have a minimally invasive equivalent. The benefits can be remarkable for many procedures. In the right hands, minimally invasive surgery is safer and has numerous benefits, many of which are heralded as the future of health care.

Proven Benefits of Minimally Invasive Surgery
- Less pain
- Fewer infections
- Shorter hospitalization
- Lower risk of needing subsequent surgery*
- Earlier return to work activity following surgery
- Lower medication use during recovery
- Cost savings from the above benefits

* subsequent surgery for postoperative hernia or bowel obstruction

Choice of procedure matters. But minimally invasive surgery is only performed by *some* surgeons, and the distribution of surgeons trained in these newer techniques is random, reflecting the happenstance of where one was taught. Curiously, big academic medical centers tend to be more behind the times than some large, non-university hospitals. Big academic centers are more often controlled by an old-guard patriarchy, making nimble purchasing decisions and shifts in practices a challenge. Acquiring the latest technology can get lost in committees, becoming as bureaucratically fraught a decision as an act of Congress.

Conversely, community hospitals are more likely to have efficient purchasing of new technology, with the freedom to buy whatever their surgeon wants. The result is that the laparoscopic revolution in America was a non–university hospital phenomenon that began in community hospitals and still thrives there today. I noticed this when I first attended a national meeting of the laparoscopic surgery society and didn't recognize a single presenter as an academic heavyweight. Instead, they were all doctors from larger community hospitals that pride themselves on rapid uptake of the latest minimally invasive equipment. Competition from a sector of medicine outside of the mainstream has produced one of

medicine's most important recent developments. Local can sometimes be better, even more cutting-edge, than big and famous.

The question for patients is: How do you know your options?
How can you find out about having a body part fixed or removed
using one of the safer operations with much lower complication
rates? For the answer, I turn to Judy Moore.

Judy beat the system. A pleasant schoolteacher from South
Carolina, she went to a leading cancer center for evaluation of an
abdominal tumor that appeared unexpectedly. After an hour on
Google she got an appointment at one of the nation's leading cancer centers. There, she was told that her tumor needed a large
open operation. Having already seen the minimally invasive description of the operation on the Internet, she came to a surgeon
who specializes in minimally invasive surgery and inquired if he
could do it laparoscopically. The surgeon said yes. She had it
done, saving her the added pain, risks, and scar of the open operation. Days later, she was back to teaching in South Carolina.
Her googling paid off.

A hysterectomy is the second most common operation performed in the United States, behind only its cousin operation,
the C-section. Roughly one third of women will have a hysterectomy by the age of sixty. Yet half of women who get the procedure
will have the bigger open operation rather than the minimally
invasive version. How does that happen? Well, let's just say that
their doctor holds their hand and leads them down the road
of the bigger procedure with more risks. Many doctors don't offer the minimally invasive procedure, or simply advise against
it. Best practices emerge and only gradually and randomly evolve
from local adoptions to uniform practice nationwide. With a bit of
transparency about best practices, local disparities would quickly
disappear.

Gynecologists who do laparoscopic hysterectomies are outraged
that half of hysterectomies in the U.S. are still done through a
big, open, disfiguring operation with higher risk of infection, all
because some doctors don't offer laparoscopy. Dr. Joe Edwards, an
ob-gyn in Savannah, Georgia, says that most of the doctors in his

community simply like to do it the old way. He and another doctor in the area are the rare exceptions; they do the straightforward procedure through a few small incisions followed by Band-Aids. Despite the radical benefits, many ob-gyn doctors won't do it that way themselves because they don't know how, and they obstinately refuse to refer to a competitor, regardless of the increased risks to the patient. But with respect to the broader surgical community, the more invasive the procedure, the higher the rate of infection, pain, scarring, hernias, longer hospitalizations, and need for reoperation. Dr. Edwards has become so frustrated with this disparity that he started an online ob-gyn 101 health blog for patient education.

Women's groups have argued that to withhold less invasive procedures is worse for women and is a manifestation of sexism, e.g., men are more likely to recommend a mastectomy than a lumpectomy. There may be a measure of truth to this.

It is true that only a fraction of all patients end up with the less invasive surgical option. Here are some estimates regarding the disparity of which patients get minimally invasive procedures:

Percent of Patients Offered a Minimally Invasive Procedure

Prostate surgery	90 percent
Appendectomy	60 percent
Aortic aneurysm repair	50 percent
Hysterectomy	50 percent
Colon removal	25 percent
Pancreas surgery	10 percent

Not all doctors fail to disclose all the options to patients, or don't refer when they should. In my hospital rotations, I met terrific doctors who were honest to the bone. I saw pockets of strong collegial teamwork, doctors who would refer a patient without hesitation if it meant better care (or lower risks) for the patient. Great teamwork like this comes about when doctors and nurses feel they are able to speak freely with one another and stay friends. Everyone is happier that way. It usually occurs at hospitals where doctors are salaried and there are no giant bonuses for racking up more operations or treatments.

One of the Hopkins survey questions asks, "At your hospital, is priority given to what's best for the patient?" The differences among hospitals are dramatic, some being strongly committed to doing what's best for the patient while, in others, employees report that decisions are rarely made based on what's best for the patient.

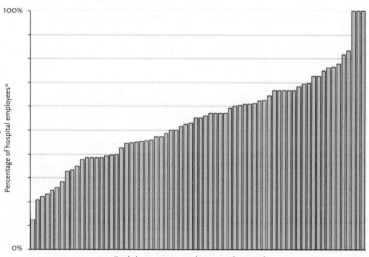

Each bar corresponds to one hospital

*Employees per hospital who report "priority given to what's best for the patient"

If the famous politician and actress described earlier had walked into a surgery department with great teamwork, instead of seeking surgery the old-fashioned way, the senior doctor might have said, "You are a candidate for minimally invasive surgery, which has a better result. I don't do it—I'll introduce you to someone who does." They could have had their procedures with a small incision and a camera and gotten back to work much sooner, with less pain and risk.

No Sheriff in Town

Medical care varies widely within our county's best hospitals. And modern medicine is not the standardized discipline most people think it is. It certainly is not the standardized discipline I thought it would be as a premed student. Our system's virtues have broken down to the point at which whether you get a minimally invasive versus large open operation depends on surgeon "style" (with the patients unaware). Take, for example, a patient with prostate cancer. That patient's treatment could be:

- Radiation
- Radiation plus surgery
- Surgery done open
- Surgery done with a robot
- Observation with no treatment
- Proton-beam therapy
- Any combination of the above

Is this the freedom of the "art" of medicine—or the chaos of subprime real estate before the crash? High dollar rewards for getting patients make doctors and hospitals reluctant to refer them to the highest-quality provider or hospital. In the case of prostate cancer, some doctor practices have bought radiation machines and make a profit from each treatment. It's not surprising that most of their patients are recommended radiation.[2]

In the years that have gone by, I have seen many other patients receive substandard, dangerous, sometimes deadly medical care. Still amazed at how this could be, I became a listener. I would listen as celebrities, politicians, and CEOs—the crème de la crème of America's moneyed and educated elite—would share with me the stories of their care. What they revealed was that they were buying their health care on promises based on rank hearsay or pure public relations jargon that would send any doctor or medical staffer into fits of laughter. One patient boasted to me that his doctor was the best because he had operated on a U.S. president. Another patient, a prominent accountant in my community, told me how much trouble he went through to get a surgeon who had operated on President Reagan. "If he was good enough for Reagan, he's good enough for me," he told me.

I didn't mention to him that most surgeons in D.C. knew President Reagan suffered from central-line complications caused by a line that was improperly put under his clavicle. Central IV lines should never be placed under the clavicle during a chest trauma: Every surgeon knows that as a routine standard of care. Then, amid concerns over a possible complication of accidental puncture, the president was subjected to open-lung surgery to ensure that the bleeding stopped. Many surgeons in D.C. who know the true story believe that Reagan may not have needed his surgery.

CHAPTER 6

Navigating the System

Picking a Doctor

By now you are no doubt thinking, How do I find the best doctor to treat my condition? Keep in mind that there are two types of doctors required by the average person: proceduralists and diagnosticians.

Proceduralists

Proceduralists do one operation or set of procedures and embody a new yet increasingly common phenomenon. Today, many doctors aspire to be known for doing one thing well. The ultraspecialist voice on a clinical dilemma is revered and respected in the culture of medicine. Doctors like to have a niche area in which they are *the* authority. Further fueling the fire is a reimbursement system that financially rewards doctors. Put simply, a doctor who can create a factory-style mass production of procedures is going to be a rich doctor. While this sounds cold and impersonal, this assembly line of health care has an upside for patients.

While the conveyer-belt style of operation introduces the problem of appropriateness of care and runs the risk of dehumanizing procedures, it does address an issue that has plagued modern medicine: the lack of standardization. Institutions that do more of a procedure have fewer mishaps, and doctors who have routinized a given treatment with dedicated teams are more likely to work in harmony.

Provided the procedure is the appropriate one, the team has likely seen every possible surprise associated with it. Their experience can ensure added safety. Efficiency and safety go way up with support staff who pass the surgeon the correct instruments, who are familiar enough with the procedure and its complications to watch for early signs of procedure-specific problems, and who are familiar with how to defuse them. In short, the same thing that makes "procedure factories" offensive might be what makes them high quality. Now imagine what type of doctor would be so driven to develop and command such a factory. A compassionate listener? Or an ambitious technician? Therein lies the reason for the frequent disassociation between warm personalities and quality care in procedures.

The landscape of modern medicine is actively being revised by an explosion of new proceduralists specializing in new areas of knowledge (and not even doctors can keep up with what the new specialties are). When I recently asked for an ENT (ear-nose-throat) specialist to look at a patient of mine in the hospital who developed hoarseness, the consultant saw the patient and then came up to me and said, "I'm an ear guy . . . You need a throat guy." I was shocked at the degree of carve-outs within a specialty. But then again, my field has done the same. When my team at Hopkins operates on an abdominal sarcoma cancer that has grown into the kidney and adjacent blood vessels, three surgical teams are involved to perform the operation in sequence. My surgical oncology team and I operate on the cancer part up to the kidney, then we call the urologist to remove the kidney, then we call the vascular team to remove and reconstruct the blood vessel. If there is a wound complication, it may be managed by a wound specialist.

Procedures in America are increasingly specialized, and the range of operations any surgeon performs is getting narrower each year. So if you hurt your hand, don't just find an orthopedic surgeon: Be sure to ask for a hand surgeon. And, as always, feel free to get a second opinion before having surgery.

While many proceduralists are well-known for streamlining

patient flow, no one has mastered it like the Cleveland Clinic's Dr. Toby Cosgrove. He organized a highly skilled team of surgeons and other specialized assistants to routinely perform several open-heart operations each day. Setting up his patients in adjacent operating rooms so he can jump from room to room, he comes in after the patient is under anesthesia and departs to the next room after completing his last stitch. His dedicated, teamwork-style surgery earned him the admiration and wonder of his peers and the hospital administration. Hailed for his exceptional outcomes, Dr. Cosgrove is now a legend for his low complication rate. You want his team. Many doctors seek him out for their own heart operations. In fact, his success creating a culture of teamwork and safety resulted in the Cleveland Clinic asking him to be its CEO, a role he holds to this day.

In the hospital, we jokingly refer to such highly specialized procedure masters as (procedure)-ologists. We call knee specialists kneeologists, and we call ob-gyn doctors who specialize in delivering babies birthologists. While such jargon is informal, it underscores how we doctors have come to think of other procedure-focused doctors. If someone had asked Dr. DeBakey, "How many spleen operations have you performed in the last year?" he or she would have been understandably frightened away by the answer. And if someone had asked a health professional what Dr. DeBakey is known for, he or she would have learned that he is a heart bypassologist.

Diagnosticians

Diagnosticians are doctors who figure out what is wrong. An effective diagnostician is a good listener with a compassionate spirit who spends a lot of time with you in order to crack the case. Unlike pure proceduralists, among whom there is no correlation between warm personalities and quality care, diagnosing and managing medical conditions is a different art. A high-quality diagnostician does tend to be marked by a warm demeanor and an approachable bedside manner. To find a good diagnostician, you have to shop around. Hospital employees can often tell you who they are.

Sometimes health plans limit your choices, making it hard to get to the right doctor. The best bet is to meet with a doctor and see how well you interact. When a patient tells me his or her doctor doesn't listen well, it is often a doctor I know doesn't have a good local reputation. Most negative feedback will correlate to those who may not be high quality. (Online reviews such as those posted on zocdoc.com or yelp.com cannot speak to a proceduralist's technical quality, but they can indicate which diagnosticians are good and which hospitals have a good service culture. Of course, ratings based on only a few reviews can be unreliable, but those based on hundreds probably are reliable.)

If your diagnosing doctor doesn't listen to you, move on until you find one who does. Studies show that in a typical doctor visit, the patient is interrupted after an average of eight seconds. That doesn't necessarily mean your doctor is a bad person. Doctors interrupt for a reason. We are trained to tabulate "hard symptoms" to solve "cases." Hard symptoms are what we are writing down while you are talking. Hard symptoms are things like fevers, vomiting, and right-upper quadrant abdominal pain (a triad characteristic of an instant gallstone diagnosis). Hard symptoms are terms we can look up in our textbooks and make instant sense of. We are trained to abstract a list of them to come up with a unifying diagnosis. As a way to be efficient, we can sometimes reduce a patient's malady to a list of hard symptoms. Conversely, we doctors tend not to be as comfortable with "soft symptoms." When patients tell us they feel tired or "blah," we might tune that out, because, quite frankly, those words don't fit our diagnostic algorithms and we like to do things by the book. When the symptoms don't match a plausible medical explanation, there's a temptation to throw up our hands. Cracking a case with soft symptoms can be frustrating, especially when we are required to see more and more patients in an hour.

I like to let patients talk for ten to fifteen minutes about everything. I won't lie: It can be painful, especially in the middle of a busy day, to listen to patients go on about what their brother-in-law's cousin thinks is the cause of the problem or how their dog is really suffering because of the ailment. However, oftentimes I will uncover something medically relevant amid verbose descriptions of how a patient was watching TV with Grandma. A small clue like "and I often sit on the couch after a meal when I get pain in my right side" can be a subtle clue of a gallbladder problem. This is why listening skills directly translate not just into polite doctoring but good doctoring. It allows a doc to be an effective disease investigator. The best diagnostic doctors I have known at the nation's best hospitals are the best listeners.

When you buy a car, you probably ask someone you know who is knowledgeable about cars to assess your options. You get a second opinion. I highly recommend getting a second diagnostician involved for a second opinion whenever the stakes are high. In general, patients are afraid to get second opinions: Some patients think it's rude, and there are financial disincentives that discourage it. A health plan will sometimes not pay for one, or it can be difficult to schedule. But when the stakes are high—as they often are with big procedures, conditions with wide variations in care, and difficult cases with no diagnosis—it's worth it. I encourage it among my patients, and even offer to run their case by my partners on their behalf. Remember that when an insurance company does not allow a second opinion, what it really means is that they won't pay for it. It's still legal for a patient to exercise his or her right to a second opinion. We live in a free country with a private health care system. You can always make an appointment with any doctor in the United States and pay out of pocket for a consultation. The highest out-of-pocket charge for a consultation would range from $120 to $400 if you bring your own records and films and don't need tests repeated. When further testing is recommended, be sure to ask what the incremental benefit is, since it can sometimes be avoided. Doctors generally assume insurance is footing the bill, so we have a tendency to order tests liberally. If we know the patient is shouldering the cost, we exercise more restraint.

Second opinions are always possible in America, even when you are admitted to a hospital. When your health is on the line, don't take chances with your life and wellness that you wouldn't even take buying a car.

The Bottom Line

One take-home message from the Shah's operation is that experience with a specific procedure or condition trumps any big title, honor, or medal. In finding a good proceduralist, the doctor you want is not necessarily the head of the department or the doc with the most academic accolades: *You want the person with the most experience in treating your specific condition.*

For example, if you need a hip operation, choose the surgeon who has done a lot of hip operations. If it were me, I would choose a hip surgeon who does a hundred hip operations a year over a general orthopedic surgeon who does five hundred total general orthopedic operations annually, but only ten of them hip operations. If you want to know how to get this information, that's simple: Ask. More relevant than any other screening tool is the question "How many cases of this type does this doctor see per year?" There is no law against a doctor divulging how many of a certain procedure he or she performs. If the doctor can't or won't divulge this data—or flounders when you ask—there's probably something amiss. A doctor who has a great reputation and is repeatedly performing a procedure with great outcomes will almost always be happy to tell this to a prospective patient.

Conversely, if I were looking for a diagnostician, I would want a compassionate listener. Someone who would let me talk. But I would still want the doctor with a lot of experience with my condition. Similarly, if I needed more empathy than medicine, I would value a doctor with a good bedside manner, a doctor who knows how to heal with words. Often the only way to find these doctors is to ask around (especially medical staff), or simply to meet with a doctor and see if the two of you communicate well together.

Health care is increasingly becoming an industry of unique disciplines of study. As medical knowledge expands, procedures are becoming super-subspecialized. Take eye surgery. Some eye surgeons now specialize exclusively in surgery of the retina, cornea, or lens. I even once met one of these docs who only operates on a part of the eye I didn't even know existed. Patients lucky enough to find him will be getting the highest-quality operation on their eye and the best chance of regaining their sight.

Insist on the Stats

Hospitals are sitting on treasure troves of data about how many of each operation they do each year. A transparent health care system would make the information public, preferably right on the web, so that people could use it in choosing their care. Coupled with how well hospitals perform, what their culture scores are, and how often their patients bounce back from complications, this information would make our free market in medicine functional. We don't want a free market that blindfolds the consumer, or in which competition is allowed to take place only on grounds of which billboard, granite lobby, or accessible parking lot seems most attractive. Insurance companies leave quality selection entirely to us; for them, it's about nothing but who's the cheapest. Without data transparency, competition will continue to be about all the wrong things, frustrating consumers and payers alike.

Consumers are starving for good data that is user-friendly to understand. One large study found that *quality* of care is people's biggest concern in choosing a health plan. It ranks well above low cost, the range of doctors they can choose from, and the range of insurance benefits.[1] Businesses and insurers might also find it in their own best interests to actively assist people to find the best medical care. Because long-term, good health costs less.

A few states, such as Minnesota and Massachusetts, have begun to require hospitals to reveal how many procedures they perform, by type, each year, for the public to use in deciding where to go for care. But for the vast majority who seek medical care, it continues to be either very difficult or impossible to find this data. The statistics are either not collected because hospitals have no incentive to collect it, or the data is collected and highly guarded. Without guidelines and controls, any reported data might also possibly be massaged. Regardless of the reason, hospital volumes are generally not publicly available. If they were, you'd be more informed in choosing your medical care. Some states have instituted a Patients' Bill of Rights. Having access to this kind of information should be considered a basic right for anyone dealing with the medical system.

CHAPTER 7

Tap the Power of Patient Outcomes

GETTING GOOD CARE CAN BE A complex maze that confuses even the savviest consumers. At some point in their life every American will choose a doctor, yet few have the information to choose wisely. Sure, magazines put out their annual "best" lists, but the fact is, these lists are based on poor information and tend to be heavily biased. Most people don't know these lists can be based on hospital nominations, and for some magazines, the criteria are not transparent. Popular magazines are good at picking up on new rumors and trends, but not as good at doing the time-consuming research to evaluate hospitals.

In 1895, Dr. Ernest Amory Codman graduated from Harvard Medical School and became an intern at Harvard's Massachusetts General Hospital. There he was flabbergasted at how the medical profession did not keep track of patient outcomes, nor did the physicians discuss their mistakes openly to instruct other doctors how to prevent them. Enraged, he watched patient after patient harmed by the same common errors. A technically superb orthopedic surgeon himself, he was later invited to join the Harvard faculty, where he had notable achievements in the field of bone cancer (a "Codman tumor" of the bone cartilage is still in medical textbooks today). But while Codman was a cancer surgeon extraordinaire, he believed that doctors could save many more lives if they learned from their patients' outcomes in a standardized way. He instituted the country's first internal peer review conference, called a morbidity and mortality (M&M) conference. Codman also lobbied hard for the hospital to keep track of every patient's end result and keep registries so that doctors could learn from prior patients. He wrote about "the common sense notion that every hospital should follow every patient it treats, long enough to determine whether or not the treatment has been successful, and then to inquire, 'If not, why not?' with a view to preventing similar failures in the future."[1]

But his ideas to track patient outcomes were not welcome at Harvard. The doctors there were most enraged by his proposal to hire doctors based on merit instead of on what connections they had and by his proposal to evaluate surgeon competence through peer review. Despite his strong national reputation, Codman was pressured to leave and was ultimately shown the door at Harvard.

Still determined, Dr. Codman went on to start his own hospital, which he called the End Result Hospital. There, he created a card for each patient that documented their preexisting medical problems, their current ailment, what was done, and what the end result was. Most important, the card would record any medical mistake and lesson learned in the care of a patient. Dr. Codman was very open about the fact that of hundreds of patients admitted to his hospital, one third of them had suffered from a medical mistake, a rate he believed to be par for the course in American medicine at the time. The registry of lessons learned was a teaching tool for his staff so they could make care safer. He also believed that the lessons learned should be made available to doctors everywhere, and that information on a hospital's overall patient outcomes should be made available to the public.

Dr. Codman's ideas for making health care better caught the eye of other forward-thinking medical leaders. Dr. Codman worked with Dr. Edward Martin, a Philadelphia gynecologist, to help start the American College of Surgeons. Soon after, Codman led the organization's hospital standardization program for national accreditation, and later started the first national bone tumor registry. But there were many political and logistical barriers to Dr. Codman's effort to measure patient outcomes on a large scale. He was ahead of his time and the medical establishment resisted

his innovations. As a result, after Dr. Codman's short-lived movement, medicine continued as a largely secret business. Ironically,
Harvard's newly created outcomes research center at Massachusetts General Hospital is now named the Codman Center for
Clinical Effectiveness in Surgery after its rejected pioneer.

Historically, knowledge of who the best and worst doctors are
has been confined to doctors' lounges and closed risk-management
meetings. However, a new generation of performance measure-
ments has matured that threatens to shake up the complacent
system we now have.

Take, for example, this new metric of health care quality: ninety-
day readmission rates. For the first time in history, computers can
track patients who are readmitted. This wasn't feasible previously,
as computer systems for different institutions had no way of "talking" to each other. Thus a patient who left hospital A and was readmitted to hospital B was considered to have no complications by
hospital A. Now all these patients are captured in databases that
generate a readmission rate for each hospital by condition (internally called "bounce backs" in medical jargon). Coupled with the
average length of the hospital stay for that condition, a consumer
could look at the numbers and figure out which hospitals have the
best track record and which hospitals kick their patients out too
soon with little guidance on follow-up care.

To get readmission rates under control, some hospitals devised
a discharge "hand-holding" plan, giving every discharged patient
an instruction sheet with a list of medications to take, and how. It
listed frequently asked questions to help patients with their recovery. Patients also were sent home with a hotline number to call if
they experienced problems at home. And before leaving the hospital, patients chatted with a nurse who explained what they might
expect in the coming days, so the patient knew what symptoms
would be considered normal or abnormal, and what might require
a call to the hospital for advice versus a trip straight to the ER. This
simple discharge-instruction hand-holding alone was considered
revolutionary.

If readmission rates were made fully public—not just the secret property of hospitals and insurance companies—positive

repercussions for society at large would reverberate through the health care system. A hospital's ninety-day readmission rate benchmarked to nationwide averages is a powerful performance marker that, if publicly reported by medical condition, also might revolutionize quality of care.

Seeking accurate ways to measure patient outcomes has long been the holy grail of health care reform, the starting point for fixing our broken health care system. Everyone wants patient-outcomes data, but no one seems to know how to get it. Mark Porter, a leading health economist at Harvard Business School, says the problem with the traditional business model in health care is that competition is generated over costs, not value. Costs and value can only be evaluated relative to outcomes. Porter's recommendations have been widely praised by politicians of both parties, but little has changed.

Economists and politicians alike all say health care reform needs to begin with measuring outcomes. But their hesitation to require this relates to concerns about the immaturity of the science of measuring outcomes. We lack a uniformly accepted definition of what a "good" versus a "bad" outcome is. An operation might be a success, but if the patient later dies, can it be attributed to a failure of the earlier care or not? Second, it is hard to monitor outcomes. Doctor-reported outcomes are notoriously biased in all studies, e.g., "I've never had a complication, to my best recollection." Third, monitoring outcomes independently costs money. Hospitals are paid more for operations that result in multiple complications than for operations that have none. So they have no financial incentive to invest in prevention or to monitor anything that might reflect poorly upon them, might get them bad press (by admitting they have a problem), or that requires them to do a lot of extra work. Finally, outcomes often don't account for how complex a patient's case is. We doctors rightly get angry when a crude ruler is used unfairly to measure our performance. Not surprisingly, metrics with no adjustments for inherent patient risk or complexity have also caused some doctors to shy away from treating higher-risk patients.

For years, doctors have opposed such data gathering, fearing that it will be misinterpreted and fail to properly adjust for how sick their patients really are. All of us that practice medicine agree that measurement of patient outcomes must factor in patient case complexity. Doctors who take on more high-risk cases shouldn't be penalized for having worse outcomes. The reverse is also true: Doctors who cherry-pick the healthy shouldn't be rewarded for discriminating. High complication rates for surgeons whose practice is composed of mostly high-risk and complex patients might very well be misleading. They might also create bad doctor incentives to start doing things to subtly rig the data (it's been done before). This dilemma has paralyzed health care reform for decades and stymied policy makers. Until now.

A new generation of doctors has been stepping up to the challenge. They've partnered with their peers and specialty associations to create ways to measure hospital performance tailored to their respective specialties. In my field of surgery, an impressive group of doctors, eager to advance the state of medical care in America, began a Manhattan Project–like effort, embarking on what was known as the National Surgical Quality Improvement Program. Most members of the group had studied the veterans' health system in the 1980s, a period in which the government was threatening to shut down all U.S. Veterans Administration (VA) hospitals, which were getting a bad reputation. Dr. Shukri Khuri and other doctors developed a complex mathematical formula to adjust complication rates for a patient's preexisting medical conditions.[2] They used a consensus to create strict definitions of what constitutes a complication, and they created a program to ensure that the stats get collected fairly. The program trains independent nurses at each hospital to collect key information on patient outcomes and their preexisting risk factors. Weighing each preexisting condition differently and accounting for its severity, the complicated formula accurately predicted the degree of adjustment needed to make comparisons fair—at least by doctors' standards.

Thus, an eighty-six-year-old patient with diabetes and heart disease had an expected complication rate different from a sixty-five-year-old who had only heart disease. The formula factored in everything doctors knew to be important, plus everything that statisticians found affected outcomes. The mathematical model found that while patient outcomes at VA hospitals as a group were much worse than at other hospitals, when adjusted for how much sicker the veteran patients were, VA hospitals were equal to private hospitals. Developed uniquely by doctors (and now overseen by UCLA's Dr. Clifford Ko and the Cleveland Clinic's Dr. Michael Henderson), the formula has had unprecedented credibility. It has been highly praised by doctors and was even adopted by the nation's largest surgeons' association, the American College of Surgeons (ACS), to compare patient outcomes across hospitals.[3] It refined the outcomes-measurement method, using expert groups to create strict consensus definitions of a complication. An independent nurse was also given full access to records and the right to contact patients and review cases and enter any complications into a database.

With the independent nurse protocol to collect patient outcomes, traditional pitfalls in data collection were whittled away. This achievement in itself is a milestone, equivalent in the field of health outcomes to landing on the moon, given doctors' reticence at having their outcomes assessed by anyone. The independent nurse goes over the data for detail, screening charts, checking lab results, and calling the patient to see if a complication occurred. (When only physicians report patients' complications, the data can be orders of magnitude off due to underreporting.)

The ACS method was the first to measure patient outcomes in a way that doctors agreed was fair. The Society of Thoracic Surgeons and other powerful doctors' associations followed in parallel, developing their own specialty-specific ways to independently and fairly collect patient-outcomes data nationwide. To date, these and other national registries collect outcomes data hailed by doctors as indisputable, and their success in providing meaningful data back to participating hospitals has led to even more widespread participation across the United States and even around the world over the past few years. In short, these national registries represent a treasure trove of valuable information.

Finally. A way to accurately measure patient outcomes had arrived!

But not for the public. The data is locked and sealed tighter than

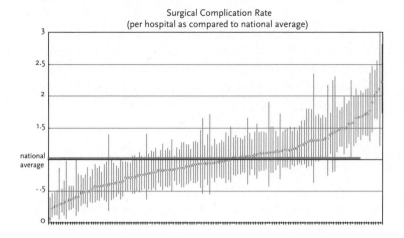

Complication score determined by observed to expected outcomes. Y-axis figures represent scores' relation to national average, with some hospitals reporting a rate twice the national average.

Fort Knox. Hospitals don't want you to see it. In hospital speak, we call it "sensitive data," available only with hospital names removed. So I can tell you that some hospitals have four to five times the complication rates of other hospitals—but I can't tell you which hospitals they are. I can publish here what I am allowed to: the range of health outcomes by hospital with the hospital names removed from the graph. Suffice it to say, like the employee-survey results, the findings are dramatic. And, like the employee-survey data, all hospitals measured are prestigious and respected in their communities.

To put this graph into words, some hospitals have *average* complication rates radically higher than others, even after the numbers are adjusted for hospital size, demographics (urban versus rural), and patient complexity. As the first description of the quality disparity among American hospitals that can be believed to be reasonably accurate, it a milestone in the science of measuring quality. It's a tool so powerful, it could force hospitals to awaken from hibernation and get serious about making care better and safer.

The independent measurement program has now been adopted at hundreds of U.S. hospitals on a voluntary basis. In the spirit of transparency, a few brave, innovative hospitals in this program are now planning to make their results available to the public. Depending on the public's appetite for this information, such a trend could grow quickly, resulting in a second landmark achievement—all hospitals responding to the demand to be transparent.

Two Surveys, One Pattern

Dr. Bryan Sexton and I were working on scoring our survey of safety-culture data in adjoining offices when the ACS graph of patient-outcome scores was released. As soon as I saw it, I shouted, "Hey, Bryan, get over here!" He came over. We gawked in amazement—the safety-culture data looked just like the patient-outcomes data (see next page). You could have superimposed the two graphs. It was as if one explained the other.

Even graphs of specific survey questions, such as *Would you have your own care at the hospital in which you work?* had the same distribution as the graphs of complication. So did a hospital's average employee response to the question *Is management responsive to my safety concerns?* We later found that mathematically, too, the graphs were very similar in slope and range. It was a study dying to be done and a study for which the results surprised no one. Just take a look at the resounding similarity in distribution of safety attitudes and surgical complication rates by hospital.

My own clinical experience, and the data, point to the fact that good teamwork and a good safety culture prevent errors and lead to better-quality care. I've never met a doctor who disagrees. The same is very likely true outside the field of medicine. When Bob Herbold surveyed his employees at Microsoft, he found that attitudes correlated with performance.[4] By the same token, if you were to study the culture of teachers in a public school system, or administrative assistants in Fortune 500 companies, those who report a respectful work environment with good workplace communication are sure to have better results due to the better workplace culture. I also have no doubt that data about public school

Operating safety culture by hospital

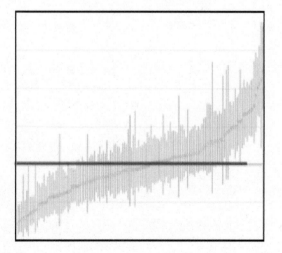

Each bar corresponds to one hospital

*Employees per hospital reporting good safety climate

Surgical Complication Rate

performance and corporate performance is more readily available than the same types of data on health care outcomes.

Several hundred hospitals worldwide have now used the safety-attitudes questionnaire. Each hospital's score is very telling, predicting medical mistakes as well as overall quality of care. Naming the hospitals would be groundbreaking. At the same time, caveats must be heeded—all scores are just snapshots that would have to be kept up to date in real time to be useful. Still, with this level of transparency, the quality of the nation's health care system would surely improve radically. To know the complication rate for a standardized hip surgery at each of one's local hospitals would be revolutionary, just as reporting mortality rates for heart bypass surgery revolutionized that procedure in New York State.

Transparency and accountability are crucial values required for anything to work, whether in government or business. Citizens have learned to ask for transparency from Wall Street and Washington. We need to ask the same from hospitals.

PART II
The Wild West

CHAPTER 8

Impaired Physicians

I WANT TO COME BACK TO AN eye-opening experience I mentioned in the introduction: I was sitting in an auditorium full of surgeons when Dr. Lucian Leape, a renowned Harvard surgeon, asked us to raise our hands if we worked with a doctor who was unsafe to be practicing—and every hand in the room went up. Thinking over Dr. Leape's question sent the faces of Hodad and Shrek flashing through my mind—my own personal collection of incompetent surgeons I've worked with. Marveling at all the raised hands, I quickly estimated that there must have been some three thousand malpracticing doctors out there related just to this audience.

Evidently, I wasn't alone in having witnessed profoundly bad medicine. Overwhelmed by the audience's unanimous response, I sat there, bewildered. In fact, when I was slow to raise my hand in the initial seconds after Dr. Leape's question, a senior surgeon sitting next to me, his hand held high, looked at me in amazement and said, "Son, you don't know of any?"

"I can think of at least one," I mumbled as I tardily raised my hand.

On further consideration I thought, This is crazy. I figured that each one of these dangerous doctors probably sees hundreds of patients each year, as any doctor typically does. This would put the total number of patients who encounter the dangerous doctors known to this audience alone in the hundreds of thousands.

Who's standing up for those patients? I thought. They probably have no way of knowing that their doctor is impaired.

As I listened to Dr. Leape talk about secret addictions and other common impairments, I realized that he wasn't just talking about doctors who simply have poor skills or bad judgment. This was an entirely different problem. He was talking about doctors affected by dependence problems and other physical and mental impairments. That's when the problem of impaired physicians struck me as nothing less than a public health crisis. I did some more math. If, say, only 2 percent of the nation's one million doctors are seriously impaired by drugs, alcohol abuse, or other major impairments (and most experts agree that 2 percent is a low estimate), that means twenty thousand impaired doctors are practicing medicine. And estimating that each one of these doctors typically sees five hundred patients each year, then ten million people are seeing impaired doctors each year.

In awe at the magnitude of the problem, I turned to the older surgeon sitting next to me and asked, "What can be done about these few bad apples affecting so many people?"

He smiled and said, "The state medical boards take care of that."

At the time, I knew nothing about how a state medical board monitors the profession. I had never heard of anyone losing their license from a state medical board's action. My only experience with state medical boards was filling out a brief application in Virginia, Maryland, and the District of Columbia to get my medical license there. The application took about fifteen minutes to complete, and the process seemed no more difficult than obtaining a driver's license.

To be sure, the vast majority of physicians are good people who make an honest effort to help others in need. Just because I'm the doctor, patients routinely trust me enough to put a knife to their skin within minutes of our first meeting. And just because I'm the doctor, patients will often tell me innermost secrets about their lives—things they'd never even tell their own spouses. Most doctors consider being a doctor to be a high honor and privilege, a job like no other, and try to treat each patient as we would our own mother or father. No doctor is infallible, but most of them are committed professionals who hold themselves to high standards.

Yet there are also grossly impaired physicians, doctors with horrible skills, hazardous judgment, ulterior motives, or who suffer from substance-abuse or other problems that make them dangerous. Society ought to be able to deal with this better, not sweep it all under the rug. Doctoring is a stressful profession with easy access to drugs, so it's no mystery why doctors have substance-abuse problems. In fact, rates of serious substance abuse and psychiatric disease among doctors are actually higher than that of other professions with similar educational background and socio-economic status.

For anyone who works at Hopkins, this subject hits close to home. If you were to ask any doctor, "Who was the greatest doctor in American history?" he or she would probably say William Halsted or William Osler, early-twentieth-century contemporaries who were the pillar surgeon and general medical doctor, respectively, of the original Johns Hopkins Hospital.

Halsted is considered by many to be the father of American surgery. He promulgated the concept of safe surgery, invented many operations, and introduced residency training to the United States. The first chief of surgery at Johns Hopkins, he is credited with many surgical firsts, including the first radical mastectomy for breast cancer and the introduction of surgical gloves—before that, doctors operated with bare hands. The Halsted clamp (a hemostat) is still used in nearly every operating room in the world.

While a surgeon in New York, desperate to find a way to make surgery less painful for his patients, Dr. Halsted experimented on himself (and his colleagues) with cocaine as an anesthetic, feeling that experimenting on himself was more ethical than experimenting on a patient in a much worse position to assess the risks. It worked. Clinical cocaine in combination with ether furthered the fields of anesthesiology and surgery, allowing more radical operations to be performed.

So Halsted was a hero. But his cocaine experiments had a dark side. Halsted and his colleagues all became addicted. During a time when little was known about drug dependency, Halsted was discreetly hospitalized in Butler Sanatorium in Providence, Rhode Island, where, trying to cure him, doctors simply converted his addiction from cocaine to morphine. He was released, but with his New York career over, Halsted joined his friend William Welch at the newly opened Johns Hopkins Hospital. At Hopkins, Halsted would quietly and methodically revolutionize American surgery.

Halsted functioned at such a high level, it is hard to believe that he very likely remained an addict during all of the many years he led the Department of Surgery at Johns Hopkins. There are, however, a few clues. He'd occasionally have to excuse himself from an operation, and he was often absent from the hospital. In his diary, published as *The Inner History of the Johns Hopkins Hospital*, Halsted's colleague Sir William Osler described finding him "in a severe chill," realizing that he was still an addict. Halsted died in 1922 as a serious morphine addict—yet still a hero among surgeons worldwide.

Like many doctors, I have seen or heard of substance abuse among colleagues. When I was a student working at Massachusetts General Hospital, the chief resident committed suicide by injecting himself with potassium—a solution kept on every hospital ward. Throughout my career, I have known doctors who were clearly burned out. I myself took a summer off after my training before starting my faculty job, expecting only that it would be nice to spend more time with family and friends and enjoy the summer. That summer, by stepping away from my work, I realized that I was incredibly burned out and didn't know it. It took the time off for me to appreciate it.

A 2009 study published in the prestigious journal *Archives of Internal Medicine* found that 31 percent of doctors are burned out and 51 percent of doctors wouldn't recommend the profession to one of their children.[1] That's some serious stress. Another study by Drs. Charles Balch and Julie Freischlag asked detailed questions of eight thousand U.S. surgeons about their lives and found that no fewer than 40 percent were burned out, 30 percent screened positive for symptoms of depression, and 28 percent had mental-quality-of-life scores below the general population norm.[2] When I heard about these results, I went through all the stages of grief in ten minutes (denial, anger, bargaining, depression, and acceptance). If the great Dr. Halsted himself had struggles pulling at him, it's reasonable to believe that they still exist in medicine, especially with the added stresses of our complex system. In my original calculation estimating the magnitude of the impaired-physician problem, I estimated that 2 percent of doctors are impaired. However, based on Halsted's life and what I've seen in my career, I agree with others that 2 percent is a drastic understatement of the true incidence of impaired physicians.

Dr. Leape's axiom is that every doctor knows at least one other doctor who is too dangerous to be practicing. He validates this axiom at scores of his lectures, by unanimous vote. After one of Leape's talks, I asked other doctors in the audience to describe impaired doctors they knew. Doctor after doctor had a horror story. They would tell it so fluidly, with a broad smile and a chuckle; it was clear it had been told many times before. Other doctors gathered round would then chime in eagerly with their own examples. Such chat fests can even turn into contests over who worked with the craziest doctor. Calling home, I tested it on my father, who is also a doctor. He had his own tales cued up and ready to go. Fascinated, I began asking every doctor I met—in every specialty—for tales of misconduct. Everyone had a story, or two or three.

Days after Dr. Leape's lecture, I bumped into a good friend who works as a cardiovascular anesthesiologist at a highly reputable New Jersey hospital. I asked him the magic question: Did he know of a dangerous physician who should not be practicing? Before I even finished asking, he began to describe a colleague who was one of four heart surgeons at his well-known heart hospital. This surgeon had six consecutive deaths during routine bypass surgery. Half the surgeries of his last ten surviving patients took several hours longer than the norm, often requiring the patient to be put back on the heart-lung bypass machine after having come off of it.

One time, right after this notoriously bad surgeon's run of six deaths, my friend was administering anesthesia for him. In front of all the operating-room nurses and technicians, the patient asked my friend before going off to sleep, "Is my surgeon a good surgeon?" The operating-room staff froze as their eyes popped out of their heads. They stared at my friend to see how he would deal with the direct question. "He's one of the four best heart surgeons we have here," he said with a smile. Luckily for my friend, the patient didn't follow up with, "And how many heart surgeons do you have here?"

Having inside knowledge about a risky doctor while trying to comfort his patient in preparation for surgery is a dilemma every health care provider knows all too well. I asked my friend if he ever thought about reporting this surgeon to someone. He laughed and asked, "Like who?"

The hospital administration loved this young heart surgeon, who was making a financial killing (pardon the pun) off his work. The senior partners were very protective of him as the youngest member of their group—after all, he took most of their weekend calls for them. He covered their holiday shifts and happily tended to whatever the senior surgeons did not like to do, such as operating on their obese patients for them. They cut the young doc tremendous slack whenever his complications were discussed at a peer-review conference, saying a patient's death was attributable to some extenuating patient circumstance. (That's right, they'd blame the victim.) "He was a smoker." "His kidneys must have been bad to start with." "The calcified plaque on his arteries made them particularly hard to sew." My friend listened to all these excuses offered up in conference. As an anesthesiologist who had to work every day with the surgeons sitting in the peer-review conference, he decided to keep his mouth shut.

Such internal peer reviews are a little like the Russian parliament under Stalin. No matter how much discussion there is, the result seems foreordained. At these internal peer-review conferences, complicated cases are reduced to biased two-to-three-minute summaries, and doctors who might raise probing questions are well aware that they can pay a heavy price for challenging their peers. Like many health professionals, my friend didn't like the safety culture in his unit, but he was no dummy. He knew that whistle-blowing could not only hurt his career but also fail to accomplish any meaningful change. At most institutions at which I've worked, I've witnessed the rare occasion of a doctor bravely challenging another doctor about substandard care only to later face major internal political blowback. I've even seen a few vocal doctors leave a hospital under pressure by the "incumbent" doctors in power there. It's easy to say that doctors should speak up, but being overloaded with work and performing complex surgery is stressful enough. When it comes to peer-to-peer confrontation at the workplace, our survival instinct guides us to retreat to a haven of neutrality: We don't need partners' anger and resentment to boot.

Hospitals sometimes fire doctors who speak up, sending a powerful warning to the medical community at large to stay in line. As I wrote this book, I learned of another whistle-blower sacked by her institution. Kiran Sagar, sixty-five, a prominent cardiologist who has trained hundreds of doctors in reading echo (ultrasound) studies of the heart and who was one of the first female cardiologists in Wisconsin, was studying an issue she is passionate about: misinterpretation of heart-echo tests by doctors, a problem endemic in many U.S. hospitals. By formally studying procedures at her own hospital, she found that the quality of the interpretation of echocardiograms varied widely depending on the doctor reading them. At a national cardiology conference, she presented her findings that in total 29 percent of heart-echo interpretations are incorrect. She concluded with a suggestion to develop more standardized methods to interpret echos and to initiate a quality-control mechanism to prevent this important heart test from being misread. You would think that a patriot who brings attention to an important medical problem would be rewarded for being a patient advocate. Exactly the opposite happened. She was instantly fired by her hospital (Aurora St. Luke's Medical Center in Milwaukee) despite a long, prominent career.[3] Tragically, her highly publicized firing over her study sent yet another shock wave reminder to medical professionals everywhere: Expose medicine's dark side of doing business and risk your own career.

Doctors and nurses know of docs who are reckless, but it takes moving a mountain to do something about it. Not reporting incompetence among peers is part of medical culture and has been for centuries. Medicine is poorly policed. Getting fired takes an action so egregious or offensive to hospital administration that I have only seen it happen twice among all the hospitals in which I've worked and trained.

How about the national doctors' associations? Can they police their own kind? As a member of several, only once have I ever heard of a program that tried to address impaired physicians, and that effort never picked up steam. After asking around, it became clear that the only time that a doctors' association would ever consider taking action against a doctor was if a state medical board had already done so. Hungry to grow their membership and collect annual dues, doctors' associations are historically passive when it comes to policing doctors (the AMA is actively recruiting to increase its membership, which has now declined to 15 percent of U.S. doctors; membership costs $420 a year). Policing doctors is a job so messy, no one wants to do it. Except, of course, in sending out dunning notices for thousands of dollars in membership dues each year.

So who is in charge of policing medical care in America? Not the FDA—they approve medications and devices as safe. Not Medicare—they just pay the bill for seniors and police billing fraud. Not hospitals—they profit from incompetent medical services that only breed more hospital services. Not the American Board of Medical Specialists—they simply give out certificates for passing certification exams. And doctors' associations view their function as just running forums for medical education, and lobbying for higher Medicare payments for doctors.

Every organization, institution, medical association, and hospital administrator that I have asked has told me that policing physicians is the real responsibility of state medical boards. So let's examine the role of state medical boards in American medicine.

State Medical Boards

Consider California. The Medical Board of California, like all others, is responsible for licensing and disciplining physicians. On three different audits conducted during the 1980s, the California auditor general found that the board wasn't doing its job.

Apart from that announcement, no further action was taken. The board went eighteen years without another audit until 2003, when University of San Diego Law School professor Julie D'Angelo Fellmeth became the medical board enforcement monitor. Then she blew a whistle. Testifying to a Senate committee in 2008 after years of trying to sound alarms, she said the Medical Board of California routinely "failed to promptly remove from work physician participants who tested positive for prohibited substances."

The board had five out of five failed audits. Still, rather than address the substance abuse among its staff, it instead decided to terminate its physician substance-abuse program completely— claiming that running the confidential program to support and monitor doctors with drug, alcohol, or mental problems was inconsistent with its mission. Julie D'Angelo Fellmeth was let go. The Medical Board of California then went on doing whatever it does about impaired physicians—which is to say, not much. (Though some medical-board members, along with hospital associations, promptly busied themselves lobbying for more doctor pay during health care–reform debates.)

Within a few months after we doctors graduate from medical school and fill out some simple paperwork, we receive a state medical license by mail. This license is as easy to abuse as it is to open the envelope it comes in. The license legally allows us to do anything in medicine. But unlike with a driver's license, you can screw up royally yet never lose your license to practice medicine. Even doctors in rehab who test positive for illegal drugs or are arrested can keep their licenses and continue to diagnose, prescribe, and operate as before. Unbeknownst to the public, surgeons can be arrested for driving drunk or stoned and then go into surgery the next day. A doctor might not be able to legally drive his car to the hospital, but once he gets there, he can open up your chest for surgery. A known alcoholic surgeon in my residency at Georgetown Hospital once came to work drunk to see a bleeding patient at night. The nurses and I watched on in awe.

Alan Levine is a soft-spoken gentleman with a big smile who worked for the inspector general of the United States, overseeing medical boards. "They vary widely," he says, referring to the state boards, "mostly serving the interests of their stakeholders— doctors." Some states let you look up a doctor's disciplinary record. Other states don't. If a medical board ever conducts an investigation—a relatively rare event—it tends to be weak. And I have never heard of a state board making a call to a witness, let alone conducting an on-site hospital investigation.

Boards do publish lists of doctors who settled a lawsuit out of court. Of course this is distorted data, because unfounded law-suits can be common. Nearly all doctors will experience a lawsuit at some point in their career, and teasing out the ones with merit can be difficult. Some lawyers seem to encourage any patient who becomes disabled to sue, hoping they get lucky with an empathetic jury. Even a life-saving amputation by a good doctor can prove difficult to defend for hospitals. Juries sometimes will hold a subpar hospital against the individual doctor, even if this is un-just in the particular doctor's case. Hospital lawyers therefore tend to settle before entering a courtroom stacked against them. Given the risk of a large potential payout, hospitals also calculate that it's cheaper for them to settle these types of cases out of court. In fact, hospital lawyers go to court on average only once for every ten to twenty lawsuits brought, opting to settle the rest.

Some state medical boards do the cheapest possible research— they just make a count of out-of-court settlements. Insurance companies are the only ones to use this data, in order to hike malpractice-insurance rates that might force a doctor into early retirement. My state, Maryland, puts doctor information online. My disciplinary record profile reads:

Malpractice Settlements (If there are 3 or more settlements of $150,000 or greater within the past 5 years): **None**

How comforting.

So, now, what do you know about me? Probably nothing new. Even if I had three settlements, it may not be an indicator of any-thing if all three were frivolous. I've actually never had any, but if I did have a couple, my lawyers would probably stretch the third one out so that three together didn't span five years.

In short, even this public data isn't strictly honest or even useful. You might expect medical review boards, instead of releasing
misleading stats, to actually investigate problems involving impaired physicians and do something about them. But, they don't,
or do so only rarely.

Moreover, Alan Levine says, states don't communicate with
each other. Surprisingly, state medical boards don't investigate
most of the doctors they license even by conducting a computer
search of the National Practitioner Data Bank, a centralized, U.S.
Department of Health and Human Services–housed list of all
doctors who've been disciplined, suspended, or have lost or settled a lawsuit against them. Being in it may not mean you're a bad
doctor, but it does raise a flag.

I have asked state medical boards why they don't query the national data bank before they issue a doctor a medical license. I have
been given many excuses ranging from limited resources to "It's
not our job." But my favorite excuse was that they could not afford
the four-dollar-per-doctor fee to query the data bank. So the state
board can't afford a four-dollar query, but it can afford to hunt
doctors down for annual licensing fees. (In ten years of practice in
Maryland, I will have paid my state medical board $3,000 to keep
an empty file on me, and a certificate; I have dropped my D.C.
and Virginia licenses to save on the expense.)

One doctor investigated for impairment in Massachusetts applied for an Illinois license so he could move his practice there. The
Massachusetts Board of Registration in Medicine was asked by Illinois if he had any issues. Massachusetts replied that no suspen-
sions or disciplinary actions had been taken. This was true, since
Massachusetts didn't have to disclose the ongoing investigation,
which could go on for months or years. So the doctor went on to
work at the Marion VA hospital. This loophole almost seems like a
gambit by which one state gets to pass on its lemons to other states.

William Heisel, a national health-journalism fellow with
the University of Southern California, did a national study of
state medical boards. Heisel found that many states funnel doctors guilty of fraud and sexual abuse to vulnerable patient
populations—namely poor communities, addiction-treatment

centers, asylums, and prisons. One Maine doctor, criminally convicted of defrauding Medicaid, was required by the state medical board to "treat 15 percent of indigent patients without charge until he becomes an approved provider for Medicare and Mainecare," the state of Maine's Medicaid program.[4] So the poor get bad doctors sicced on them.

If state boards and national doctors' associations aren't stepping up to deal with impaired physicians, what about hospitals and their staff? Big-name physicians who get large referrals bring hospitals volume. The more revenue a doctor brings in, the weaker the hospital's incentive to look into local allegations.

The information in the National Practitioner Data Bank is also known as the national "blacklist" of doctors. I obtained a deidentified copy of this data to research patterns of dangerous doctors and repeat offenders jumping states. I had always thought that someone could look me up in the database to see if I was in there, but to my surprise, I learned that the public has absolutely no access to it. The data set I was given has the doctors' names deleted. The only groups that can query the list are a state medical board or human resources department doing a background check. Not the public. Ironically, sex offenders' names are broadcast to the community when they move into town, but doctors who lose their licenses in one state because of sexual misconduct with a patient are shielded by name in the database if their license is later restored or if they continue to practice medicine in another state.

The lack of cooperation between hospitals and state medical boards resembles the problems of the Roman Catholic Church—another nontransparent and unaccountable system—which failed to remove dangerous child-molesting priests, opting instead to reassign them to other parishes. A 2011 report by the group Public Citizen found that the small fraction of doctors disciplined by their hospitals are often not reported to their state medical board. Between 1990 and 2009, there were 10,672 doctors with hospital disciplinary actions pending against them. More than half were not reported to their state medical boards, including 220 doctors who had lost medical privileges on an emergency basis due to the immediacy of the threat to the safety and health of the public.[5]

By and large, dangerous doctors still see patients. If their hospitals or state medical boards do go so far as to slap their wrists, the doctors can simply skip town and set up a shingle somewhere where no one knows them, and their new patients will not know of their problems. Meanwhile, Alan Levine's office, which was dedicated to the fair oversight of doctors, hospitals, and state medical boards, has been eliminated.

In a story on state medical boards, the *Washington Post* concluded:

> When medical boards are faced with how to handle substance-abusing doctors, they often use rehabilitation as a substitute for discipline. In the Washington area and across the country, physicians who test positive for drug or alcohol abuse are monitored, and sometimes they must agree to therapy or other steps. But rarely are they banned from practicing. . . . Even when doctors enter residential treatment programs, they often retain their licenses to practice.[6]

Impaired physicians are a small minority of doctors who are very destructive and difficult to police. Knowingly or unknowingly, they cause a lot of harm. State medical boards are sometimes aware of them, but look the other way. Standards for doctors are local and vary widely state by state. They should be national. Airline-pilot standards, on the other hand, are national standards. Imagine if an airline pilot who was fired from one airline for flying while drunk could simply get a job with another airline without any other consequences. Or that a pilot who was barred from working in one state for endangering passengers could just get a flying license in another state. Would you feel comfortable getting on a plane? The aviation industry knew that relegating flying standards to the state purview would result in some states with high standards and others with low standards—the nature of state diversity. Realizing how this would hurt public safety, the FAA decided to oversee standards (e.g., how many flight hours of experience a pilot must have to fly certain sizes of commercial planes, how long pilots may fly without sleep, and how pilots should be disciplined for being impaired). Having a similar set of minimum national standards for doctors would allow state medical boards to adhere to some general principles, such as not granting licenses to doctors who lost a license in another state. It's one common-sense solution that would decrease the impact of public harm by a small group of impaired physicians.

Doctors with Tremors

The aviation industry got it right. They understood that for safety standards to properly protect the public, the standards needed to be national, not local. That way dangerous pilots can't hop from state to state if they get in trouble. Aviation also polices the competencies of older pilots, screening them with regular physical exams for vision loss and physical impairments that might diminish their ability to fly safely. The FAA removes older pilots who lose their vision, their judgment, or their ability to communicate rapidly. After all, pilots are in charge of people's lives—but aren't doctors, too? Doctors work until they die—sometimes into their eighties and nineties. One surgeon mentor of mine told me, "You will find me in the hospital every day until I get chest pain or a stroke. In which case, just take me down a few floors to the emergency department and tell them to do everything."

We doctors don't like to retire. It's a fact. As a whole, we are the least likely profession to retire at age sixty-five. Why? We love our jobs. Dr. John Cameron, seventy-six, is our chairman of surgery emeritus at Hopkins. In the operating room next to mine, he continues to operate all day, five days a week, which is more than when he was the chairman. When he gets excited talking about a great operation, he frequently tells those of us younger surgeons, "When you love your job, you never have to work again for the rest of your life."

Another reason some doctors don't retire is that medicine comes to define their entire self-worth. It can be so consuming, doctors might not ever develop other hobbies. Even if we do, nothing is better than being respected by colleagues and patients for one's professional wisdom and skill. With each passing year of being a doctor I find the respect I am given increases, and the more I love what I do. It's a good recipe for never letting go. But the result is that there are many older physicians in practice. According to one recent report in the *New York Times*, one fifth of doctors are over the age of sixty-five and many practice well into their seventies.[7]

While there are some reasonable concerns regarding aging doctors, I in no way advocate removing privileges from a physician based purely on age. Older physicians are great, especially when they love their jobs. I would love to have a senior, seasoned expert as my doctor if I had a tough diagnosis. However, I would *not* want a geriatric doctor if that doctor is physically impaired. Some aging doctors have vision problems or memory loss and may not realize it. Others don't know how to use or interpret newer tests like CAT scans. These impairments can be overshadowed by their dedication and confidence. I, for example, want to practice medicine as long as I am able, which I hope is decades into the future. I can't imagine not being there for my patients or ever giving up the thrill of curing disease with surgery. The problem arises, though, when and if my health prevents me from operating safely and I don't recognize it.

Yet at every hospital I have visited, there is always some staff's ganglike effort to push out some very old doctor whose skills have deteriorated to an extreme but who refuses to quit. Often, these senior doctors will be relegated to tiny offices without a window or secretary in the effort to send them a not-so-subtle message. Others have their pay and support staff cut. One world-renowned hematologist was forcibly escorted out of the hospital by security because he just kept showing up even though he had been taken off the payroll.

Nearly every doctor can name a doctor who needs to retire but won't—impaired doctors in their nineties who refuse to leave the office even when they are no longer being paid. Why do we have this problem? The reason is there are no rules. Only a very few doctors' associations, legislatures, or insurance companies have focused on standardizing ways of ensuring that doctors older than seventy take physical exams testing for memory loss, blindness, and tremors as a condition of employment.

Dr. Karl Serrao at Driscoll Children's Hospital in Corpus Christi, Texas, believes patients deserve a high bar for their doctors. He is leading an effort at his hospital to require that doctors over seventy years of age take annual exams for vision and memory as a condition of employment. In my opinion, Dr. Serrao is a hero for the kids at his hospital. For doctors who still perform surgical procedures, basic tests of manual dexterity and screening against encroaching tremors should be required. These screening tests would weed out those doctors who are simply not realizing the extent to which they are growing impaired and give those who are still fully functional the freedom to practice without the stigma of ageism.

Impaired in the Nest

In the medical school I attended, and in the ones in which I've taught, one rule always holds true—90 percent of the students perform well and 10 percent struggle. Among those who struggle, some simply have trouble absorbing the information. Others are just too hungover, drugged up, or dealing with too many untreated psychiatric problems to get through the workload. Each year, this group amounts to a couple of students in each class. When they show up to class after a night of partying, the rest of the class is thinking the same thing: "How would you like him or her for your doctor?"

No one in my large medical-school class actually dropped out—the school makes sure that hardly ever happens. But these outliers skimmed the trees. A sardonic phrase that cropped up whenever med students started to worry about underperforming was "C=MD."

Bo was one guy we all worried about. He and his friends were often absent from class. They'd get other students' notes and "back exams" (old copies of the tests) and simply cram the night before. The next morning they'd stumble into the exam hall with two number-two pencils and regurgitate the answers before crawling home and sleeping/hibernating for two consecutive days. It was a formula for graduating that many students dabbled with but some consistently lived by. There were no skills tests, no psychiatric evaluations, no attendance sheets, and no accountability.

As I progressed through medical school, I realized that we were a diverse group—not unlike my college classmates. Out of approximately two hundred students, some had substance-abuse problems, a few were generally regarded as dishonest, and one had a serious psychiatric illness. *All graduated.* In my surgical residency, out of the twenty-five residents in my program, two had substance-abuse problems, four had career burnout, and one had a serious psychiatric illness. None got help. *All graduated.*

After we doctors graduate from medical school, the government, via state medical boards, pretty much gives us a pass to do whatever we want. The only request from the boards is that we submit some paperwork demonstrating that we participated in CME (Continuing Medical Education), which can consist of a few quizzes in the back of a medical journal or attendance at a Caribbean medical conference.

In summary, after I graduated medical school and got my license based on a 70-percent-or-higher passing score on my board exam, I was literally licensed to do anything in medicine—perform brain surgery, prescribe chemotherapy, remove varicose veins, or do electric-shock therapy for psychiatric disorders. With this government pass, I can administer unproven vitamin remedies through an expensive intravenous infusion or I can do well-established chiropractic manipulation.

I can legally do anything. In fact, some varicose-vein removal centers in the United States are run by former ob-gyn doctors and others by psychiatrists; they were doctors looking to do something different and took a weekend course to learn how to do it. Putting aside how I get paid, I can do whatever I want in medicine with little to no accountability.

Admirably, some hospitals have started taking the bold step of having their "mishaps" reviewed by doctors at another hospital—one that has no business or political conflicts of interest. This new "external review," easily done via teleconferencing, eliminates the many barriers to honest feedback and makes peer-to-peer review more formative and objective, at times humbling even the most senior of doctors. More hospitals should participate in external reviews. The discussions are educational and often introduce new ideas. A few hospitals have even begun reviewing complex patients in this forum before major treatment recommendations are made. State medical boards and professional doctors' associations could be an ideal vehicle to facilitate such reviews between hospitals.

At minimum, state medical boards should communicate better, coordinate with hospital investigations, adhere to minimum national safety standards, and disclose the name of any physician who has a license revoked because of the category type "immediate threat to the safety and health of the public." Moreover, disclosure to patients of what training a doctor has completed and public reporting of board-certification status is yet another important step toward a transparent marketplace where consumers can make the decision about whom to trust.

CHAPTER 9

Medical Mistakes

ON MY FIRST DAY OF WORK AT the Johns Hopkins Hospital, I met Dr. Peter Attia, a surgeon as physically fit as any athlete I've ever met. A brilliant young doctor, he regularly wowed the staff with his athleticism. And he showed it. A muscular, tan, thirty-four-year-old guy shaved bald to minimize resistance for swimming competitions, Peter had less than 1 percent body fat.

Not only was Peter an Olympic-level swimmer, but he was also a brilliant laboratory surgeon/scientist who had just done two years of dedicated research at the National Institutes of Health (NIH), working on a cure for cancer. Peter was the hospital's most popular role model for medical students and young surgeons in training. I had heard a lot about him before I met him in the Hopkins cafeteria on my first day at work.

"You're the new guy from Georgetown!" he called out to me with a broad smile and an outstretched hand.

Joking about the bad hospital food, Peter and I hit it off. He asked me what my research focus was going to be at Hopkins. Given his hard-core scientific achievements in the laboratory, I was apprehensive to admit that I did "soft" health-services research. I replied timidly that my research was in the area of "medical mistakes," figuring he'd have little interest. But he instantly stopped chewing his food and his expression turned intensely serious. He whirled around to pull up his scrubs top, exposing his back. It was hard to look at, even for me, a surgeon. His *GQ*-perfect V-shaped back was disfigured by a large surgical scar.

"They operated on the wrong side," he said.

A simple back operation had gone awry. A few years before I met Peter, he had an episode of back pain, quickly saw a doctor who told him he needed surgery, and had it done right away. But when he woke up from the surgery, he could tell something wasn't right. As soon as he was in the recovery room after surgery, he could tell that the exact same pain was still there, plus he noticed that he had a new foot-drop paralysis on his opposite side. Not only did the surgeon go in on the wrong side, but a nerve was injured, affecting his good side—a problem that luckily resolved months later. The mistake led to a painful and debilitating cascade of procedures that to this day prevent him from playing most sports.

"It was the worst year of my life," he told me. His experience seemed to be a humbling lesson for both of us, and an untold commentary on modern medicine. Talking through what happened also seemed to be partly therapeutic for Peter. He never sued the careless surgeon, and asked me that I use his case as a wake-up call to our profession. He explained that since his medical mishap, he turned to swimming because it was the only sport his back could tolerate. He thanked me for working on preventing medical mistakes and man-hugged me as if we were brothers.

As I would sit in conferences over the next year and hear of patients who sustained similar avoidable mishaps, I would sometimes glance over at Peter and note how much the accounts bothered him. He later told me that hearing about mishaps was a painful reminder that his disability could have been prevented. In his own doctoring, I noticed that when Peter heard or sensed that a patient was not properly informed about the care he or she was to receive, he would sit with the patient for an hour, or however long it took, to explain things. He became known for his heroic moments, taking things into his own hands to ensure good patient care. Peter worked hard to be totally transparent with patients, even though it was exhausting to take the extra time to do so.

Even though, in my opinion, Johns Hopkins is one of the safer hospitals in the country, tragic mistakes still happen there. And when Peter saw them, he became visibly frustrated with doctors who regarded surgical complications lightly or blew off their mistakes without asking the question, "How can this be prevented next time?"

Just one year short of completing his seven-year surgical-training program, Peter Attia left medicine altogether. Having been the victim of doctors who did not communicate *what* they were doing or the *risks* of what they were doing, he left feeling disillusioned by what he saw on a day-to-day basis. Peter described feeling that modern medicine was too frequently dishonest with patients, at times understating risks and overtreating patients as a matter of reflex. It was a reflex so common and so ingrained that it was hard to appreciate from within the profession. But Dr. Attia knew all about it—and its consequences, firsthand. Every day as he went to swim, he was reminded of modern medicine's collateral damage.

Being in the medical-errors field has decreased my threshold for shock. A *New England Journal of Medicine* study concluded that as many as 25 percent of all hospitalized patients will experience a preventable medical error of some kind.[1] Almost everyone I talk to has a story about a friend or family member who was hurt, disfigured, or killed by a medical mistake. Even me.

My research partner, Peter Pronovost, lost his father due to a medical error when Peter was in medical school. My medical partner, Dr. Patrick O'Kolo, lost his younger sister due to a medication error. My best friend's mom had her breast removed unnecessarily because she was mistakenly told she had stage-three breast cancer. After her procedure, her doctors told her the original report had a mistake—she had only had stage one and hadn't needed a breast removal after all. My grandfather died at age sixty from a condition called urosepsis, a preventable infection following a surgery he didn't even need. My brother has a wide scar on his back from his stitches popping open after a skin mole was removed; he thinks it was unavoidable bad luck, but I can tell the surgeon used stitches too weak to hold the skin together. My cousin worked with a cardiac surgeon and witnessed countless deaths from an impaired physician. I myself was misdiagnosed with a knee problem in medical school. This almost resulted in my aborting plans to be a surgeon, were it not for an excellent third opinion from orthopedist Dr. Eric Hume that resolved the issue after a few months of physical therapy.

Doctors are not surprised when they hear that Andy Warhol died prematurely of a mistreated gallstone at the age of fifty-four, or that *Saturday Night Live*'s Dana Carvey had open-heart bypass surgery on the wrong vessel. John Wayne's fatal colon cancer was missed at Harvard because his doctor didn't want to inconvenience him with a rectal exam. Had he caught it, the John Wayne Cancer Institute might have gone to Harvard rather than UCLA. The singer Kanye West's mother recently went to a surgery center for a routine plastic surgery, developed a rare complication, and died.

In the case of West's mother, her surgery took place in a freestanding surgery center where there was no adjacent hospital to handle emergencies. This is now a common scenario. Patients don't know, and aren't told, that if something goes wrong, they are going to be up a proverbial creek without a paddle. When the day comes for me to have an outpatient procedure under general anesthesia, I'll do it at an outpatient surgery center connected to a hospital. Thirty-eight percent of outpatient procedures are done today from ambulatory surgery centers with no adjacent hospital. No matter how good the doctors are, that's a less safe place to be.

Gagging

Listening to Peter and many friends who have similar stories, I realized that these patients suffer not just from their botched treatments but from the knowledge that their misfortune need never have happened. For them, talking about medical mistakes is part of their healing. But our system wants to sweep them under the rug and keep them quiet. I sometimes hear egregious stories from people who preface their accounts with, "Please keep this just between you and me, because I signed a waiver saying that I would never talk about this." When a doctor or hospital does harm a patient, the settlement offer from the hospital often contains a confidentiality clause (aka "a gag rule"). In fact, in any case of gross neglect, hospital lawyers will aggressively pursue victims or their surviving family to settle out of court quickly in order to stem off a malpractice suit—provided they agree never to speak about what happened, even if one has been disfigured, maimed, or killed.

Gag orders aren't just being used on victims of medical mistakes: They sometimes appear in the fine print of the form you sign when you walk into a doctor's office. In 2011, Robert Allen Lee, a Washington, D.C., area man, developed a painful jaw infection and went to a doctor's office, where he was treated. But weeks later, after a bitter billing dispute, Robert posted this online review of his doctor on Yelp and DoctorBase:

> Overcharged me about $4,000 . . . Refuses to submit the claim to my insurance company. When asked for records to submit the claim myself they referred me to a 3rd party that wants [$268] to get the records of me.[2]

As the *Washington Post* reported, the day after he posted the review, Lee received a letter from the doctor's practice threatening to sue him for at least $100,000 for "defamation, slander, and libel" and reminded him that when he came for medical care, he signed a letter that barred him from publishing a critique. While this doctor's threat backfired because the *Washington Post* shed light on the conflict, consulting firms are touring the country adding gag forms to the papers you have to sign in doctors' waiting rooms.

I understand the value of keeping secrets when they are related to business strategies or creative new ideas, but gagging patients about their experience with medical care? In my experience as a doctor who has made mistakes that harmed patients, I have found that patients appreciate an honest conversation about things that go wrong with their care. In order to get a handle on the wide-spread epidemic of medical mistakes, we need more conversation about them, not less.

Enlightened lawyer Patrick Malone, a former hospital defense counsel, and concerned citizens Sue Sheridan and Veronica James are separately spearheading efforts to ban gag rules in settlements after medical mistakes.[3] These are people who know firsthand the long-term maladaptive effect these gag rules have on the healing process. Malone is motivated by what he saw for years in his work defending hospitals. Sheridan became active in this cause after her son developed a disease from a medical mistake and when her husband died from a misdiagnosis involving a "lost" pathology report. James led a movement in New Jersey to ban gag orders after she was pressured to sign one following a clear-cut medical mistake. These pioneers fight to protect freedom of speech from being trampled by the vested interests of hospitals. And yet many patients are not being heard. In my experience, the more we can be open and honest about the problem, the more likely we are to fix it.

Mount Sinai

Mount Sinai Hospital on Manhattan's Upper East Side was one of New York's most respected medical facilities. Its transplant center in particular was famous, having accomplished many firsts in the field for its size and stature. It was considered by many in surgery to be the best liver-donor transplant center in America, a judgment that might have even been true—in the daytime. But at night it was a different story. Chasing profits like so many other hospitals, Mount Sinai chose to shrink nurse ratios from one nurse for every six patients to one nurse for every seven. And its unsafe overnight operation relied on only one intern. (In the hospital where I trained, the staff all knew the first-year surgery intern working the night shift on the transplant service was overworked and spread way too thin.)

Tragedy arrived one night when the intern on call for transplant surgery, just months out of medical school, was in charge of covering thirty-four complex patients. She was also on call for all transplant-related patients who came into the emergency room. A fifty-seven-year-old man, former *New York Post* writer Michael Hurewitz, came in. He had altruistically donated part of his liver to save his brother's life a few days before and now was back in the hospital, vomiting blood. The overwhelmed intern didn't know how to handle it. For hours she failed to call her senior surgeons to ask for advice. Tragically, Michael Hurewitz wound up choking on the blood he was vomiting and died. After his death, the transplant program shut down. A lamentable end to an important hospital unit—all because teamwork was poor and management had no good mechanism to elicit staff-safety concerns so that they could be corrected.[4]

The errors interns make generally don't come to light. Every now and then, however, the patient is a journalist. Betsy Lehman was a *Boston Globe* reporter. She was killed by a mistaken dose of superconcentrated chemotherapy at Harvard's famed Dana-Farber Cancer Institute. A young doctor there had accidentally prescribed the lethal dose.[5] The death became a cause célèbre, and the institution nearly shut down in the wake of the high-profile tragedy. Similarly, when Libby Zion, daughter of a prominent New York journalist, died from a medical mistake committed by overworked interns, intense media scrutiny led to the passage of a law in her honor limiting doctors to an eighty-hour work week.[6] When we residents heard about these high-profile medical errors in the news, we would roll our eyes, finding it odd that these ubiquitous events only caught the public's eye when someone with a megaphone took notice.

We had deep objections to the way safety was marginalized in the giant health care system, but the alternative was not to practice medicine at all. Participating in the hazing of "being in over our heads" was the only way to become a surgeon. So we did it and deferred our deeper questions. Medical mistakes were common and the reasons we made them were many. That's why we found it amazing that the subject of medical errors only seemed to make it to the public eye when the victim was a journalist.

After the tragedy at Mount Sinai, the hospital started listening to its staff by hiring a consulting firm to talk to staff and report back to the administration (an expensive way to achieve the same ends as a simple safety survey—or even officials walking the halls and talking to the staff themselves). Mel Granick, a spokesman for the hospital, said it would eliminate the use of first-year residents from the transplant ward. He also said the hospital was committing to a ratio of one nurse for every four patients.[7] Mount Sinai responded to the medical catastrophe by making a dramatic about-face. But the problem could have been detected and solved simply by querying staff concerns earlier, or via an employee-safety survey. The fix was finally made—but too late for Michael Hurewitz.

Hurewitz's preventable death was a tragedy resulting from a poor teamwork culture, a system of poorly backed doctors and nurses spread too thin, and a management that had no good mechanism to elicit staff-safety concerns. A state investigation uncovered ninety-two complaints about Mount Sinai Hospital: seventy-five were about the liver-transplant unit and sixty-two of them involved patient deaths.[8] Again, as Georgetown residents, we were not surprised at all. On the contrary, we were members of similar setups for disaster and knew that what happened at Mount Sinai could have happened at many reputable hospitals.

There are bad doctors and impaired doctors, but the problem of doctors making repeated avoidable mistakes is a *management* problem. Not only do unsafe hospital systems allow bad and impaired doctors to keep on practicing, they foster situations in which even good doctors will make mistakes.

Given the national attention devoted to Mount Sinai's lethal error, one might expect other hospitals to take the story as a cautionary tale. Instead, as a result of new shortened work-hour guidelines, there is a shortage of trainees available to work, meaning that residents are now covering far more patients at night (i.e., they are cross-covering more patients on nights and weekends). Residents pass off pagers so often that some residents on call carry five or six pagers on their belts—one for each service they are covering. I have yet to meet an intern who doesn't think this is another ticking time bomb.

Some hospitals have done the right thing and hired additional nurse practitioners and physician assistants to help cover the night shifts, supporting on-call interns. But the vast majority of U.S. hospitals simply spread their on-call interns even thinner. Dr. David Bates, a professor at the Harvard School of Public Health and a national authority on medical errors, believes that the new work-hour policies "appeared to have no impact on safety."[9] Doctors in training today are responsible for covering more patients at night than when Michael Hurewitz died.

In many hospitals, interns are discouraged from asking senior physicians for help even when they desperately need it. Every intern knows the feeling. In fact, when I heard that this Mount Sinai intern didn't call promptly, I had flashbacks of a personal nightmare I experienced at D.C. General Hospital when twelve trauma patients rolled in on the same night. Already instilled with the warning to be very cautious about bothering seniors for help at night, I timidly called my chief resident, asking him to come down to help.

"Why are you calling me?" my chief barked.

"Because there are twelve trauma patients here, sir," I explained.

Obviously annoyed, he asked, "Well, what are you going to do for their injuries?" He was clearly angry.

"I don't know, because I've only seen two of them so far, but I could really use your help since it's just me down here," I said, in shock that we were even conversing about the need for him to come down.

To my surprise and utter horror, he then shouted, "Dr. Marty Makary, you need to learn how to get organized!" and hung up on me. He never came down.

That night I did my best to bandage, sew, and manage twelve

trauma patients with only one medical student helping me. Two of those patients died.

For Americans who don't believe in rationing care, I have news for you. I was rationing care that night. It was absolutely impossible for me and one other student to give all twelve patients the attention they required. Even worse, I was subconsciously being taught a lesson that I was not expecting to learn—beware of bothering your seniors at night. The next morning, at our morning-report meeting, I saw my chief resident. I looked as haggard as a desert nomad, unsteady on my feet, and bitter about the exchange with him the night before. My chief looked sharp and clean-shaven. With a half smile, he looked at me and said, "Good Morning, Dr. Makary. How did it go last night?" as if nothing had ever happened. After that, you can imagine my reluctance to call my chief resident on a night when I had only one trauma patient and was only in a little bit over my head.

No one should be treated like this, I would often think to myself; my peers felt the same way. About half of my coresidents considered quitting to work in a friendlier culture. Some did. A few years ago, when six out of the seven surgical interns at Harvard's Massachusetts General Hospital quit, those of us who'd survived surgical residency weren't surprised.

As interns covering vast numbers of complex patients at night, we were well aware that calling a senior doctor was like walking into a minefield. And as burnout intermittently burdened our lives, the art of not getting yelled at sometimes superseded the goal of providing good patient care. Among interns, some surgeons were well-known for not seeing their patients after surgery and for having a short fuse. In fact, the Mount Sinai surgeon who operated on Michael Hurewitz never saw him after surgery. And when I inquired among doctors who worked for him, they confirmed that this surgeon's fuse was very short.

In any industry, a management unresponsive to the concerns of its workers is a management destined to neglect safety. In the medical business, such managers are also unlikely to change their practice of having interns care for an enormous number of patients. After all, interns are cheap. Most hospitals are like the one I trained in—residents are paid close to minimum wage yet are responsible for forty to eighty patients each night (some in intensive care). To this day, these duties can continue for residents in training after they have already worked for twenty straight hours. The management where I was a resident didn't seem overly concerned with patient safety. In fact, at no point in the five years I worked there (averaging 100 to 120 hours a week) did any manager, supervisor, or administrator ever ask me if I thought my coverage duties were unsafe for the patients. When I showed up for the first day of work, I got a lecture about discipline and then was handed a pager, which minutes later started to beep with questions from nurses about complex patients I hadn't yet met.

At Georgetown, like most every hospital, the hospital administrators were hidden yet in charge. I didn't feel that management was responsive to my safety concerns, in part because I didn't even know who the hospital management was and in part because they never asked me. (After five years, I did eventually meet the head of the hospital at my going-away dinner.) Furthermore, if these administrators were out of touch with me, how much more must they have been out of touch with the dangerous and impaired doctors there?

My Error

As an intern, I managed the D.C. General Intensive Care Unit (ICU) at night. Alone. In the ICU, many patients were on breathing machines, so each night I looked at dozens of blood-gas lab results and made changes to each patient's breathing (ventilator) machines accordingly, increasing or decreasing the volume and pressure of air set to blow into their lungs as well as the percentage of oxygen in that air. The patients were tied down to the metal of their beds, or, as we say in the business, "restrained." One miscalculation could make a patient feel as if he or she was dying from too much or too little air. The patients couldn't talk. As I walked around and looked at them, I would often wonder what their eyes were telling me. Sometimes they tried to move their lips or even write something down, but for the most part I was left guessing what they were thinking—if they felt comfortable or as if they were being tortured.

It was 3:30 A.M., and I was a human zombie. I'd been working for twenty-four straight hours. In my exhausted haze, I misinterpreted one patient's blood-gas lab result and gave the nurse an order to change the ventilator settings. Suddenly, the patient couldn't breathe. She began to gasp for air, writhing around in the bed like a fish out of water. Per routine, the patient was restrained, with her hands tied to the bed as most patients with a breathing tube were. It looked like human torture; it was hard to watch. Minutes later, the nurse, seeing that the patient was in serious distress, rushed into the room. The patient was gasping and gagging as if it was her last breath. Alarms were sounding from multiple monitors. Just in time, the senior nurse acted alone and changed the air-flow settings. Luckily, that heroic move averted a "code blue"—a respiratory arrest.

The patient never recovered and died a week later due to a hospital-acquired pneumonia. I often thought, What if I hadn't made the mistake? Maybe she would have lived. It bothered me and affected my mood for a year. On the outside, I was a proud surgeon at Georgetown. Privately, I felt shame and guilt. While I'll never know if I indirectly killed that patient because of my mistake, after about a year I had to talk to someone about it. Over a late-night drink at a bar with my two closest friends in residency, I shared my story as they looked on with comforting smiles.

"Mart, that's peanuts compared to what I've done," one friend said.

The other laughed and said that he had made the same mistake, in the same ICU, but in his case the patient died instantly. We went on to share how we should never have been working forty straight hours, how wrong it was for us to have no supervision, and how "thin" we were covering fifty or sixty critically ill patients by ourselves. They pointed out how much safer the hospital would have been if it hired a dedicated nurse or physician assistant to help us out at night, to check on urgent matters and help us with the inevitable scenario of having two patient emergencies at the same time. Instead we often felt that we were in over our heads, left with no choice but to subtly ration care at night.

"Mart-dude. It's the damn hospital's fault!" Chris said in disgust. He went on to argue that the system had killed the patient, not I.

While I'd always believed in personal responsibility, I found comfort in thinking my mistakes were in part the product of a flawed system of delivering medical care. I realized that hospitals create or eliminate safety hazards based on their incentives, be they profit, a good public image, or a mission to give high-quality care.

Hospital systems have improved since then, but only slightly. Unsafe hospital systems with thin doctor coverage abound, and trainees regularly work twenty-four consecutive hours. When anchor Trace Gallagher asked me about the study showing that one in three doctors admitted to having made a mistake that killed a patient, I publicly said it sounded plausible but privately thought the statistic was way too low for certain fields, like mine—surgery.

Every health-services researcher knows errors are common. I'm constantly meeting people who want to tell me how their mother got a wrong diagnosis, or their grandfather was mistreated for cancer. People seek me out to tell me their nightmare stories about medical errors. Other doctors are never surprised. They might be outraged at a doctor's sloppiness or feel the patient should have been referred—or they might see themselves making the same mistake. In my specialty area of pancreatic diseases, I have found about half of the patients with a pancreas problem have been inappropriately evaluated before reaching me.

Medical mistakes are not only far more common than they should be—they are a devastating cost burden on our health care system. Consider the total economic burden of one mistake over time: The University of Chicago took organs from an HIV-positive, Hepatitis C–positive donor patient, a fact they did not detect, and gave the organs to four different patients who were clean. Those four patients now all have HIV and Hepatitis C, costing themselves and society a lifetime of HIV and hepatitis medication. They also risk losing their organs and needing another transplant, since those infections threaten organ transplants. A multimillion-dollar mistake and one that irreparably scarred the lives of those patients involved.[10] Even expenses for "below the radar" mistakes are high, such as ICU care and radiographic studies for patients being monitored following a medical mistake. These mistakes constitute the vast majority of medical errors in health care. By and large, hospitals are paid more if there is a "below the radar" mistake, since there are more medical services to charge for. Using the *New England Journal of Medicine* report that 25 percent of all hospitalized patients are harmed from a medical mistake in some way, consider the instant cost savings of a 50 percent reduction in mistakes alone. The government disproportionately pays for mistakes, since older Medicare beneficiaries are at the greatest risk for medical mistakes and constitute as much as one quarter of the revenue for hospitals.

Health care costs constitute one sixth of our economy. Medical mistakes are a heavy tax on our society via costs that are passed on in the form of higher medical bills, higher insurance premiums, and higher deductibles. The societal cost of mistakes is also passed on to taxpayers in the form of rising Medicare costs as the leading growth driver of our mounting national debt.

When I was in training, one of my fellow residents left a metal object inside a patient's abdomen (a one-foot-long, two-inch-wide metal "aide" we routinely put in the abdomen to protect the intestine when we sew the deep layer of the abdomen closed). The patient was quietly taken back to the operating room to remove it once the error had been realized, but there was no centralized tally or national registry to keep track of how many of these events occurred that year. Today there is. Hospitals routinely collect the number of so-called never events that occur each year. Never events are things that should never happen, like operating on the wrong patient or on the wrong side of the body. Take, for example, the never event of a sponge left inside of a patient. Some reputable hospitals I have visited have told me that it occurs at their medical center three or four times a year. Medication-dosing errors are far more common never events and will be tracked carefully with new electronic health records. If the annual rate of never events per hospital were made public, then hospitals could begin to compete on safety rather than on parking.

CHAPTER 10

Ask Before You Give

Children's Hospitals

As a teenager, I always watched the Children's Miracle Network telethon. Pictures of bald kids with cancer. Newborns with cleft lips. Toddlers with muscular dystrophy limping along in pain. From the time I was in junior high, I vowed to do my part to help, organizing our key club to have a car wash to raise money for the local children's hospital. We raised about $175. As an adult, I have continued to donate to fund-raisers to support children's hospitals. Through medical school, I admired pediatricians most, knowing it takes a special person to work with kids. Children's hospitals held a special place in my heart, and the doctors and nurses who work in them still do.

But my admiration of children's hospitals as charitable pillars of our profession was dampened last year after I learned more about the ways they spend some of the money they raise, namely on growing executive pay packages. I had heard from pediatricians at one of these hospitals that the institutions do not spend wisely the millions of dollars they raise from small donors in their communities. With one of my research students, I began looking into the finances of these hospitals. In the process, we discovered that some children's hospital CEOs now make over $5 million per year, and some had perks including cars, first-class travel, country-club memberships, and special retirement packages worth millions.[1]

CEO Pay at U.S. Children's Hospitals

	Tax Status	CEO	Annual CEO Compensation (reported in 2009)
Children's Mercy Hospital of Kansas City, Missouri	Nonprofit	Randall L. O'Donnell	$5,987,194
Children's Hospital of Wisconsin, Milwaukee	Nonprofit	Jon E. Vice	$5,465,948
Children's Hospital Medical Center of Akron, Ohio	Nonprofit	William H. Considine	$5,132,104

Source: "CEO Pay Packages, Ranked By Hospital Revenue," Kaiser Health News, September 27, 2011

There is a national shortage of pediatricians and pediatric nurses in America. Low pay relative to other specialties is considered to be the leading driver of the supply problem (starting salaries for pediatricians average around $110,000). In addition, the field needs an infusion of money to address the many patient-safety issues that are magnified in this vulnerable population: Children are disproportionately affected by medication errors and disproportionately fall through the cracks in the system, problems that continue at alarmingly high rates today. One pediatrician friend of mine who works at our community children's hospital in Washington, D.C., told me that their CEO had been making cutbacks while increasing his own annual salary to $2.1 million (plus benefits). National Children's is a nonprofit organization, doesn't pay taxes, and raises big money every year from the community. I'm all for rewarding performance, but how is their performance evaluated? It's certainly not based on improved patient outcomes and lower rates of medical errors. Here was a local example of hospital management paying itself forty to fifty times more than it pays its average pediatric nurse. Digging further, I learned that this small, three-hundred-bed hospital was paying its CEO far more than the CEO of our mammoth two-thousand-plus-bed Johns Hopkins Health System. It became clear to me that executive compensation was another example of poor accountability among the leaders of our nation's hospitals.

It turns out that the local children's hospital in Washington, D.C., was not alone in feeding fat salaries to its managers. The CEO of Children's Mercy Hospital in Kansas City, Missouri, was paid nearly $6 million the same year the hospital blitzed the community with fund-raisers.[2]

Collecting Pennies

In one fund-raiser for Children's Hospital Boston (Harvard's children's hospital), children were asked to collect pennies from other children at school. This for an organization that recorded a $111 million surplus that year (2009) as a nonprofit and paid its CEO millions.[3] In other words, they collected pennies from kids and made tons of money. Hospital fund-raising is so lucrative that the hospital has 125 full-time fund-raisers—more than the number of primary-care pediatricians there. Like most children's hospitals, the reason it spends so much on such an enormous fund-raising department is that it pulls in so much money. Children's hospitals are an attractive cause—one no one would dare oppose. But where does the money go? Unconvinced that donations go directly to fighting childhood diseases, I now give my money to charities at which they do, and charities that have annual surpluses under $100 million.

Children's hospitals have it made. With a steady revenue stream of tax dollars from government Medicaid programs and a mission that seems above reproach, tax-free children's hospitals make record profits and pay their executives record salaries. Children's hospitals make hundreds of millions more dollars than full-service hospitals, which average a meager 1 to 3 percent profit margin annually. In 2009, the last year records were available, Texas Children's Hospital recorded a $275 million profit and Children's Hospital of Philadelphia (CHOP) $359 million. That same year, Reuters reported that half of the nation's full-service hospitals weren't even breaking even. Yet CHOP also got a $121 million grant from the government.[4] Few people, including donors and policy makers, know that children's hospitals are doing this well.

Hospital-executive pay escalated even through the 2008–2009 economic downturn. These CEOs aren't doctors or nurses—they're administrators. No other large, nonprofit organization in America has executive pay even in the same ballpark. Gail McGovern, president and CEO of the American Red Cross, was at the center of heated controversy when she was paid $565,000 in 2008.

Children's hospitals do good work, but some are run by administrators who do not embrace transparency. Giving is a personal choice. It should also be an educated choice. Before you pull an all-nighter at your school's dance-a-thon to raise money for your local children's hospital, take a look at its IRS filings and ask how your donation will be used. You might ask if the hospital discloses their infection rate or gags kids and their parents after a medical error. If you're not satisfied, consider giving to research foundations dedicated to curing childhood diseases.

In my opinion, if a children's hospital aggressively raises money from its community, the profits ought to be going toward addressing the health care issues facing children—not filling administrators' pockets as they increase their salaries with the same arguments we've heard from Wall Street moguls. The nation's severe shortage of pediatricians and pediatric nurses is now manifesting in growing access disparities and longer wait times for care. We have a pediatric-doctor-and-nurse-shortage crisis—not a hospital-CEO shortage crisis.

When I was in medical school, I saw my classmates consider pediatrics as a career choice, then reluctantly decide against it because they could earn triple the income as an emergency room doctor or radiologist (an appreciable difference in pay when dealing with massive school debt). As local medical centers merge and are bought by giant corporations, a common practice of some institutions is to freeze health care workers' salaries to increase hospital profits. Children's hospitals ought to be sharing their abundant profits with their workers, and making pediatric primary care and nursing a more attractive career choice by paying them competitive salaries.

For too long, no one has questioned the massive government funding of children's hospitals. Healing sick children is an unimpeachable cause, but sponsoring massive cash reserves is not. Children's hospitals' mammoth profits and increasingly lavish CEO pay suggest that government subsidies to these institutions should be reexamined. As nonprofit organizations, children's hospitals are accountable neither to shareholders nor investors. Lack of accountability alone should be cause for concern and closer scrutiny. As the recent financial crisis demonstrated, organizations that seem to be all for the public good and take billions in government subsidies, such as Fannie Mae and Freddie Mac, can sometimes also prove hazardous to the nation's health.

Corporatization

An informal poll of my friends reveals that about half of them think it is reasonable to pay hospital executives multimillion-dollar salaries, given the revenue and personnel they manage. The other half think it's scandalous. But all agree that it is unethical to raise massive monetary surpluses from local schools and charities while making cutbacks to frontline workers *and at the same time* increasing executive pay to exorbitant levels. The escalating salaries of nonprofit children's hospital executives is just beginning to become a source of public embarrassment for health care institutions. American taxpayers were outraged when they discovered they were expected to continue paying high salaries and bonuses to AIG executives. Today the nation is eager to find ways to cut government spending. Do we really want tax dollars supporting record surpluses and extravagant CEO pay in health care? We learned the hard way that however noble the cause may seem for any industry that receives billions in taxpayer funds, it still needs to be held accountable.

I was recently introduced to Pulitzer Prize–winning writer Gilbert Gaul, a seasoned *Washington Post* journalist who had been studying the children's hospital excesses in parallel to my own public health policy research team's investigation. Mr. Gaul confronted children's hospital executives and accountants about the moral dilemma of harvesting children's pennies while paying executives millions. He concluded that children's hospitals play a masterful game at arguing that donations and government subsidies don't subsidize executive pay, with rationalizations such as "column A is not column B." In other words, they utilize cost shifting.

According to *Forbes*, children's hospitals raise approximately one quarter of their revenue from donations. An executive from Children's National hospital who shall remain nameless recently appeared on a telethon begging for donations; a few months later a new organ-transplant center opened for parents to donate organs to their children who need transplants—the beneficiary, presumably, of all those hard-begged new funds. It sounded marvelous on paper. Rather than use its own surgeons or increase its own surgical staff, however, the hospital contracted with MedStar Health for adult-transplant surgeons to swoop in, remove the parents' organs, and swoop out.

Soon after the center opened, a Children's National resident, on arriving at work, took one look at one of the patients and exclaimed, "What is that?" It was one of the parent donors. He looked like Gulliver among the Lilliputians. The pediatric staff's inability to care for its new oversized patient wasn't its fault. Adult medical care was outside its trained area of expertise. The new business enterprise the administrators had embarked upon posed severe medical-safety issues. If the patient had no complications, he could sail out of the hospital in good health. But if anything went wrong, a doctor could reach into a crash cart to find only predosed pediatric medications.

Sure enough, the dad developed complications after the surgery. He was put on a breathing machine. The hospital's doctors knew only how to manage children on ventilators. Knowing they needed help, the pediatricians phoned the itinerant transplant surgeon who had "swooped out" after performing his surgery. He made a few recommendations over the phone without seeing the patient. The father's condition worsened and days later became critical. Amid an uproar among the hospital's pediatricians, the patient was transferred to the hospital where the transplant surgeon worked. Luckily, both the father and the child to whom he donated survived—that time. The situation got a lot of attention among doctors in the area and was considered to be such a breach of patient safety that Children's National soon announced the closure of this transplant program.

Why hadn't the operation taken place at the surgeon's main hospital, an established transplant center, to begin with? It was obvious that Children's National had neither the capacity nor the expertise to treat adults. Yet a richly paid CEO pushed for his commuter-transplant program without bothering to understand the medical realities or the safety issues. He did, however, know that transplant services are extremely profitable.

Children's hospitals should spend more money on making their hospitals safer, rather than on country-club benefits for their executives. Nurses, doctors, and techs have plenty of good suggestions at every hospital about how to prevent mistakes. Residents still work thirty straight hours caring for critically ill children. Hiring a few more doctors and nurses might be a good start.

If you want to give to a children's hospital, be sure to give wisely only after asking about their and a few comparable hospitals' financials and transparency. Utilize resources like the websites of Charity Navigator and Kaiser Health News to see how your pediatric center ranks. A nonprofit in good financial health should put at least seventy-five cents of every dollar earned directly into actual medical services and have the paper trail to prove it. Pick a local nonprofit who will show you exactly how your money will be used to help children, and what your money will be used to buy. Many outstanding and well-run charities who don't pay administrators $5 million a year exist; they will be delighted to specify how they intend to spend your money to help sick children.

CHAPTER 11

Eat What You Kill

The Back-Surgery Orbit

REMEMBER MY COLLEAGUE DR. PETER ATTIA, who had the wrong-side surgery on his back? Why had he had back surgery to begin with? Peter thinks it should have never been prescribed at all, and that his back pain could have been managed with physical therapy and pain control. The answer is that back surgery is one of the most profitable areas in modern medicine. The incentives to go into back surgery are so strong that young, highly trained surgeons today are choosing back surgery over brain surgery.

I routinely witness young medical students interested in fields such as brain cancer doing amazing research in residency. These talents have very promising careers in brain cancer, but as they proceed through their training, they see the high-dollar rewards for sidetracking their cancer research to become back surgeons. Dr. Michael Lim, a neurosurgeon at Hopkins, told me that for a complex brain-cancer surgery taking twelve hours, Medicare pays him about $5,000. But a short *two-hour* back operation pays a lot more. That's a powerful incentive. Stacking two or three back operations in a day instead of performing a long, delicate brain-cancer surgery would allow him to earn between $15,000 and $20,000 in a day. It's no surprise that each year, an increasing number of neurosurgery graduates are going into back surgery exclusively.

As this marketplace began to transform, stories emerged of patients who would undergo six back operations in two years, such as Ronald Johnson, a sixty-two-year-old former machine-tool operator in Portland, Oregon. The *Wall Street Journal* uncovered the scam when he was told he needed a seventh spine operation. It surfaced that he had felt progressively worse after each back operation, but he trusted his doctor.[1] It wasn't until the *Wall Street Journal* profiled his doctor's sky-high reoperation rate that the public knew to stay away from him.

In Louisville, Kentucky, five neurosurgeons put in a record number of metal implants that screw into a person's spine to add stability. In 2009, that group performed the third-highest number of spinal fusions in the country on Medicare patients. In addition to what Medicare paid them with tax dollars, the surgeons received $7 million directly from Medtronic, the company that makes the metal implants.[2] Were those procedures warranted? Who knows. But I can say with confidence that spinal fusions are in a controversial gray area. In fact, some back-surgery indications are very questionable. Conservative back surgeons maintain that degenerative disc disease (the most commonly cited indication that spinal fusion is required) does not require surgery and can be treated just as effectively with physical therapy and pain medication. However, the lure of a surgical fee can minimize the recommendation to try the long course of physical therapy and pain control first.

Medicare procedures are paid for with tax dollars. When people talk about rising health care costs, I think of the $2.3 billion a year that the government pays for this one procedure alone (a 400 percent increase from 1997 to 2011, according to a *Wall Street Journal* calculation).[3] From the standpoint of the country's fiscal health, it's clear to me that wide differences in medical care, like that of back pain, are the real driver of increased costs.

As a medical student, I worked briefly with Dr. Alexander Vaccaro, an orthopedic surgeon who specializes in back surgery. The Food and Drug Administration first approved spinal implants for fusion in 1995, sparking a surgery frenzy. Hospitals have rushed to recruit spine surgeons and build spine-surgery centers. Dr.

Vaccaro has benefited from the trend, and has disclosed receiving between $415,000 and $2.03 million in royalties from six device makers in 2009, and between $165,000 and $666,000 in consulting fees from nine device makers—as well as stock in twenty-eight companies, mostly medical-device makers. His hospital ranked fourth in the country in the number of complex spinal fusions performed, receiving about $30 million from Medicare over five years for spine surgery. Dr. Vaccaro is a pleasant, fun guy with a great smile and an open attitude. He has done nothing illegal. I don't question his clinical judgement, just the financial conflicts of interest. It's a field with few well-defined standards. And when patients come in with a bad episode of pain, they sometimes like the idea of a quick fix better than a long course of drawn-out physical therapy and pain control.

Medical research funded by interested companies often favors those companies, although it isn't always the case. I myself make it a practice never to accept industry funding for any of my research studies. Yet routinely, after one of my studies makes the headlines, these companies rush to my office to suggest funding my research. I consider this to be a kickback and don't want the temptation to bias, even unconscious bias. Declining such one-on-one grants from the industry is becoming more common in the medical community. It would be better if the industry simply paid into a fund to support objective scientific research administered through the NIH or other neutral scientific or medical organizations. Correspondingly, these organizations should be protected from commercial influences. For most medical organizations, their ties with big pharma and device manufacturers can be described as arm-locked. In fact, once when I arrived at a meeting of a large national surgeons' association, I was given a punch card when I picked up my name tag and conference materials at the registration booth. The welcomer said, "Here are your conference materials, and here is a card listing our industry exhibitors here at the conference. If you visit each exhibitor's booth they will sign your card, and if you get all exhibitors to sign your card by the end of the conference, you'll enter a contest to receive a free iPad." I told her, "I'll pass."

An Instilled Reflex: The Culture of Doing Stuff

The culture-survey question *Would you have your own care at the hospital in which you work?* not only roots out the Shreks and the Hodads, it also detects doctors who treat too much.

Treating patients is what we are taught, and many times expected, to do as doctors. It's very easy for treatment to become *over*treatment. We are wired early in medical school to do things because we can. When helping a human being enter the world, doctors are taught to first deliver the baby out of the mother. The very next thing we are taught to do is to stick a probe into the baby's rectum to take a temperature. When I was in medical school and told to do this, my first reaction was, "Why?"

"Because we can't get it from the mouth," I was told.

Is strep throat in newborns so epidemic we need to inflict a rectal probe on every newborn baby? If done a few years later it'd be considered a life-altering trauma. Later, in medical school, when I had the honor to deliver a few kids, I declined to take the temperature. I also made sure no one else did unless they could give me a reason other than "Just to know." Those babies ended up doing just fine.

Medical school is so hard, not because the concepts are difficult, but because there are so many of them. For example, knowing that gout crystals in the urine mean you prescribe the treatment for gout—colchicine—is not a "hard" concept. It's just that there are so many thousand diseases and corresponding treatments.

The best way to manage all this information is to couple things in pairs in our minds. Diseases are coupled with treatments: Cancer = chemotherapy. Abnormal lab tests are coupled with the remedy: Low potassium = give potassium, high cholesterol = give a cholesterol-lowering medication, et cetera. Tumors are coupled with the name of the operation to remove them, and so on. There is so much to learn that everything in medicine becomes an entity coupled with the thing to do for it. The result is that we subconsciously develop a reflex to react to a diagnosis, symptom, or radiographic finding with the corresponding treatment or next step.

As I participated in this mass-memorization game, I realized that what got lost was the *appropriateness* of when to treat. In fact, one time when my dad, a hematologist, was helping me study for medical-school exams, we were reviewing treatments for lymphoma. As I recited a long litany of diseases and their corresponding treatments, he interrupted me by clarifying that one treatment was only to be given if the patient could tolerate such a toxic dose. "Dad, please," I said. "We don't have to know that for the exam!" I later realized my frustration with my dad's warning marked how robotic I'd become in medical school, valuing thinking fast rather than thinking smart—something instilled in me without my realizing it.

Medicine's culture of doing things just because they can be done was most apparent to me when I was a student and spent a lot of time with an elderly patient named Ms. Banks, whom I had been assigned to follow. She had been diagnosed with ovarian cancer, a cancer with a very poor prognosis. The team was 99 percent sure of the diagnosis, they told me, based on the results of a CAT scan and her blood test. When I heard this, the coupled concept "ovarian cancer = the hysterectomy with bilateral salpingo-oophorectomy operation" spit up out of my memory bank: The conventional treatment is major surgery to remove the uterus, cervix, fallopian tubes, and ovaries. But I got to know Ms. Banks very well and she told me that she just wanted to spend time with her family and do a few more things before she died, rather than have an operation or undergo chemo. After I explained to her that she could be passing up a potential, albeit unlikely, cure, I respected her wishes and tried to communicate this at the morning staff meeting at which her treatment plan was discussed. I began the conference by presenting the case:

"Ms. Banks is an eighty-two-year-old African-American female who—"

"Has she had her biopsy yet?" the attending surgeon briskly interrupted.

I stood up and began to explain that she didn't want treatment for her tumor, so perhaps there was no need to proceed with a biopsy and MRI. Needless to say, I was shredded up, down, and sideways in front of all my peers and other attendings (the people who would evaluate and grade me). As they peppered me with questions over why it wasn't done yet, I objected.

"She doesn't want anything done," I cried on deaf ears. "Why are we going ahead with the biopsy and MRI if she is declining treatment?" I knew the MRI in her situation was not accurate to diagnose ovarian cancer and I was disturbed by the fact the doctors did not care that Ms. Banks was claustrophobic, so that being put through the narrow tube of the MRI machine would be traumatic for her. In response, the attending doctor ordered me to sedate her just before the MRI so that she could have the test.

His explanation as to why we needed to press on was so self-serving, I couldn't believe it: "Even if she doesn't want anything done, we need to biopsy to know what it shows."

Perplexed, I told them what the radiologists told me the day before, that her CAT scan was 99 percent definite for ovarian cancer. The senior attending doctor responded angrily by saying, "Ninety-nine percent isn't good enough. In medicine you need to know for certain."

Ms. Banks didn't. I even asked her point-blank, "Do you want to know what this tumor is?" Her response was, very clearly, "No." Ninety-nine percent was more than good enough for her. But by overstating the benefits and understating the risks, the doctors convinced Ms. Banks to sign a form to undergo the biopsy procedure. She was a courageous lady, but she finally succumbed to the strong push of her doctors. The informed-consent process was pathetic, and hardly informed. I could tell she didn't really know why she was having the biopsy. I knew this because her doctors couldn't even tell *me* why she needed it. But the drive for the doctors to react reflexively to her tumor by ordering a biopsy was like a train no one could stop.

Unfortunately, when Ms. Banks went in for the procedure, the biopsy needle accidentally hit a major blood vessel in the area of her cancer. Her bleeding complication resulted in an added six-week stay in the hospital that was marked by blood transfusions, multiple CAT scans, and malnutrition, since most of the time she was not able to eat because the hematoma blocked her intestine.

Those six hellish weeks turned out to be six of her last nine on earth.

Clearly Ms. Banks was not properly informed of the biopsy risk. We had foisted an unnecessary, unwanted, and ultimately harmful procedure on our patient. This was no longer a debating point to me. It harmed someone I cared about. I was called into the head attending surgeon's office to explain what happened, and I recounted my objections to Ms. Banks having the biopsy. I was told that sometimes patients don't know what they want and we need to decide for them. I thought to myself, This is just dishonest, and not why I went into medicine.

Amid a flurry of pleas to stay, I left medical school. I felt disillusioned. It seemed as if, despite all the book knowledge I had gained, nearly half of the patients I saw in the clinics had problems for which modern medicine had nothing to offer except phony names for diseases we didn't understand. The other half of the patients seemed to be sick because they were obese, smoking, or not taking care of themselves—preventable problems. I felt as though it was time to leave medicine, and I did.

I enrolled in the Harvard School of Public Health, where I discovered a great passion. I loved studying the global burden of disease, ranking health priorities, and talking about how to change behaviors on a large scale. But in the end, I missed bedside patient care. At the same time, I found great mentors who did public health, surgery, and research; were highly respected in all three fields; and were at the cutting edge of medical care. Later I went back and finished medical school so I could continue to be able to practice medicine the way I thought it ought to be practiced—with honesty.

When You're a Hammer

Another major reason for medicine's wide variations in recommendations is the when-you're-a-hammer problem. It plagues modern medicine at every level. As an idealistic medical student, I assumed there were well-accepted, evidence-based standards that govern how treatments are recommended to patients. But I had a major wake-up call when I sat in my first group conference as a young doctor. The presenter put up a CAT scan for the surgeons to weigh in on. The CAT scan showed one problem: a two-inch tumor lighting up in the middle of the patient's right liver lobe. It was most likely a tumor we call a hepatoma, resulting from a long-standing but inactive hepatitis B infection. The patient was otherwise young and healthy, without any signs of cirrhosis (liver damage). The cancer surgeons recommended cutting the tumor out. The transplant surgeons in the audience recommended a liver transplant. I was flabbergasted. Why on earth would any doctor recommend a transplant? His liver function was perfectly normal, by all the tests.

"When you're a hammer, everything's a nail," my colleague muttered under his breath.

After the conference, perplexed at the recommendation to swap out the young man's liver—committing him to lifelong immuno-suppression medication and an infection risk similar to people with HIV—I inquired further about his story. It turned out that this patient had obtained a few second opinions, including two at Ivy League medical schools, both of which recommended a transplant. But at both places the "liver expert" consulted was a transplant surgeon, not a cancer surgeon. Removing the tumor on the right side without removing the entire liver just seemed so logical to me. A liver-transplant operation alone has so many risks, including a one-in-five chance of dying in the first several years due to the body's rejection of the new organ or an opportunistic infection that notoriously afflicts transplant recipients. And the immunosuppression has a long-term risk of causing lymphoma. In terms of quality of life alone, transplant patients frequently bounce in and out of the hospital in the first few years. Also, were the surgeons factoring in the ten pills transplant recipients have to take every day for the rest of their lives (compared to none for the alternative procedure)? On so many levels, transplanting this young man seemed wrong to me and to most of my colleagues.

I called a friend who is one of a few surgeons in the country who trained extensively in both transplant surgery and cancer surgery. He explained there was a battle for turf taking place nationwide between transplant surgeons and cancer surgeons: Both claim to be liver experts. He said that each has a different perspective based on what they know how to do. He concluded by repeating what my colleague had said during the conference. When you're a hammer, everything's a nail.

The principle holds true across every area of modern medicine. Given the splintering growth of new sub-specializations in medicine today, the expression now seems to come up a few times a day when I'm talking with fellow doctors as we try to understand why certain treatments were done in the past.

Doctor as Salesperson

Stories about overtreatment among doctors abound.[4] The topic has been researched a great deal and it's clear to me that every subspecialty of medicine has its own particular tropism toward overtreatment. My own field, pancreas cancer, certainly does.

Pancreas cancer is half of my practice at Johns Hopkins. Collectively, four of us perform more pancreas surgery than any hospital in the world and have a lot of institutional wisdom on the disease. By way of background, pancreas cancer is curable only 5 to 10 percent of the time. In spite of this, we see many patients with pancreas cancer come to us after having been wrongly told there is nothing that can be done, and conversely we see many patients who are overtreated. Surgery is the only hope for a cure for pancreatic cancer. My life is dedicated to offering that hope to patients who want it. It is a choice for *patients* (with their doctors' counsel) to decide how aggressive to be in going for the cure. If a patient is highly motivated, and the tumor is removable (i.e., the patient is an appropriate surgical candidate), I would go for a cure no matter how low the odds. But ultimately the choice is in the hands of the patient. I work hard to ensure that a patient is completely and correctly informed.

However, only a fraction of all pancreatic cancers are caught early enough to qualify for surgery and a chance at a cure. The majority have an average survival of fourteen months. Pancreas cancer is perhaps the fastest-growing cancer, and chemotherapy doesn't work well. Only one quarter of pancreas cancers respond to chemo, and patients who do chemo live only about *one month longer* on average. That's right, just one month. The most favorable study of a new chemo combination demonstrates a survival benefit of two months, but the regimen is highly toxic. In fact, it's downright miserable.

Studies to support the benefit of radiation for pancreas cancer are even shakier. To study the question once and for all, a European cooperative group did a multihospital, randomized trial to examine the benefit of radiation. The trial ended early because it showed no benefit, plus some harm.[5] To this day, hardly anyone outside the United States gets radiation for pancreas cancer because of this highly cited study. However, within the United States, radiation is a common treatment.

If you had inoperable pancreas cancer, would you want to come in for chemo in the last year(s) of your life for an average survival benefit of one to two months? It's an individual choice. I love life and want to live to be a hundred, but if I get inoperable pancreas cancer, I can tell you that I'll be moving to the Caribbean and enjoying what's left of my days with a piña colada in hand and the sand between my toes. Knowing what I know about it, I definitely won't be coming to the hospital three times a week for an IV needle stick to put a toxic chemo drug in my system that could mean that I'll spend my precious last days feeling weak and nauseated.

These decisions are ultimately the patient's. But personal choice can often be contaminated by a doctor's financial conflict of interest as, in effect, a salesperson for the chemotherapy drug. Yes, doctors make a commission on the sales price of the chemo. Unlike other medications that can be bought on the free market with a prescription, most chemo medications are sold only at hospitals. If you choose chemo, the doctor and hospital make thousands more in income in the form of a markup on the drug. People need to know about hospitals' financial incentive to give chemotherapy. Of course doctors should be paid for their time, and for the service of infusing the drug for those who choose it. But the charge for the service is separate from that for the drug and you can't shop for the chemo by price the way you can with other medications. The hospitals have the storeroom keys. Hospitals own the chemo medications, and you have to pay them at whatever price they set, with whatever commission they set as the sales agent.

The conflict of interest that this nontransparent system creates is significant and rarely disclosed to patients. It has the potential to sway borderline medical decisions. Even though doctors by and large are good people, they live with the many forces pulling at them amid the day-to-day grind of practicing medicine. One of those forces is their boss or hospital administrator keeping a close eye on how many dollars the doctor is bringing in. Can we be surprised if they advocate therapies that offer more income for themselves with a marginal gain for the patient?

It's a frustration I appreciate. Once I came in at two A.M. to operate on a young girl with appendicitis. The appendix was ruptured and the operation was very difficult, taking two and a half hours. The insurance company paid me about $600 for the operation, including the three fifteen-minute follow-up visits. After a few sleepless nights like that, I can relate to doctors' temptation to find creative ways to make more money. Hospitals explicitly pressure their doctors to do more procedures and see more patients in order to make more money. One doctor I know received an e-mail from his department head that read:

> As we approach the end of the fiscal year, try to do more operations.
> Your productivity will be used to determine your bonus.

He replied, "Do you want me to start taking out normal gallbladders without stones?"

In fact, many surgeon friends I know across the country have received similar e-mails or ultimatums. But not doctors at the Cleveland Clinic. They are all paid a flat salary to encourage *appropriate* medical care. Strong tension exists between the two models of getting paid—what doctors widely refer to as "eat what you kill" versus fixed salary. On one side of the debate are institutions like the Cleveland Clinic, arguing that incentives promote bad medicine, and on the other side are compensation consultants who make a living coming into hospitals and telling them how much more money they can make by converting doctors to a strong, formulaic, eat-what-you-kill incentive plan.[6] Suffice it to say, the eat-what-you-kill plan is popular among hospital administrators, and the salaried plan is popular among young doctors looking for a job.

Given the various forces at play—the doctor's diagnose-and-treat reflex, patient expectations, and powerful financial incentives—most patients end up getting chemo and/or radiation for pancreas cancer. It's their choice, but the real question is, How are the options presented to them? I have seen thousands of patients ordered to get things done they really didn't need or want. Just like Ms. Banks. She didn't need or want her procedure. But she got it anyway because her doctors strongly urged and expected her to. She ultimately trusted those doctors to dictate what was the best thing for her to do.

Perhaps more distressing than the undisclosed sales commission and overtreating of pancreas cancer is that, in my experience, most patients are never informed that the outcome will be a meager one-to-two-month added survival benefit. One highly cited study showed that approximately half of all cancer patients received chemo or radiation treatment the same week as their death.[7] As a cancer surgeon, I think all of us in the field of cancer can recognize when a patient is very close to dying. We can do a better job of individualizing proper care while being respectful of a patient's right to die with dignity and comfort.

Cancer centers have become profit centers for hospitals, thanks to the increasing number of services they prescribe and the surcharges added to the price of chemotherapy drugs. Nowadays it seems that every hospital has an expanding cancer center. These flashy new buildings are often paid for using chemo-infusion revenues. Next time you walk into a hospital, notice how the granite lobby of a cancer center gleams in the sunlight. Then compare it to the chipped linoleum of the other wings.

The underground marketplace of medicine should be transparent for patients to see. Patients should be told all their options in a fair manner, detached from the sales pitch inherent to hospitals that use an eat-what-you-kill model to reward their doctors. Whenever confronted with a decision about your medical care, inquire about the difference in average outcomes and quality of life among the options—all these are facts that should be made plain to patients before such treatments begin.

Finally, patients would be better informed if hospitals disclosed how they pay their doctors, by the Cleveland Clinic model or the eat-what-you-kill model. Wouldn't you want to know if your hospital e-mails its doctors threatening not to pay them their bonuses if they do not reach procedure volume targets? Next time you're seeking care, inquire which compensation model is used to pay the hospital's doctors. You may be surprised what you learn.

Lucentis

Chemo meds are not just used for cancer. Ophthalmologists can sometimes use them to treat certain eye conditions. Accordingly, like oncologists, they too can get massive cash supplements for prescribing them. The *New York Times* reported in 2010 on doctors who get bonuses for meeting prescribing targets set by drug companies. The doctors sign a contract with a drug company not to talk about their kickback arrangement or disclose any details about it. The *Times* found one such bonus program for one of two drugs used to treat age-related blindness (Lucentis, price tag $2,000 per injection, versus Avastin, $40 per injection). The newspaper calculated that a doctor injecting Lucentis could earn $58,000 a year for meeting prescribing targets.[8] I'm convinced that few of the patients getting Lucentis know that drug companies pay doctors for meeting sales targets.

The range of medical fields in which this kind of incentivization takes place has never been studied comprehensively. There's no way to definitively know how many doctors are out there pushing drugs on the public unethically, with sales targets fore-most in their minds.

Some doctors' associations, like the AMA, have now required that doctors disclose commercial affiliations to medical journals when publishing and to medical audiences when speaking at conferences—but what about to patients? Recent disclosure rules are requiring that doctors report money received from drug and device companies, but the disclosure is not required to the pa-tient: It's to the government, which makes a database available to the public. While many people praise strong financial incentives for doctors, these incentives have detracted from the public trust in certain hospitals where incentives have gone too far.

Friends from the Pig Roast

During my tenure at Johns Hopkins, I heard rumors among health care professionals about too much cardiac stent surgery going on at St. Joseph Medical Center near Baltimore. St. Joseph is a reputable community hospital located about seven miles from Johns Hop-kins. I know many people who use it routinely for their care. It has a modest old building attached to two gorgeous new Ritz-Carlton-style buildings—a cancer center and a heart center that are big moneymakers for the hospital. But the safety culture was rumored to be not good there, and overtreatment was said to be rampant. We all heard the stories. We also treated some of the victims. So it was no surprise to open the newspaper one day to read the headlines about Dr. Mark Midei, a Hopkins-trained cardiologist found to have placed more than five hundred heart stents in patients unnec-essarily.[9] Doctors were shocked too—but less that it happened than that he got caught. I figured such a big exposé meant he was going to jail. But instead the doctor later just took another job at the medical-device company Abbott, a manufacturer of stents. It was convenient since Abbott knew Dr. Midei well. In 2008, they'd thrown him a pig roast costing $1,407 for placing thirty stents in a single day, what may have been a company record.[10]

Cardiac Catheterizations

Cardiac catheterization is the X-ray-guided procedure used to place heart stents by sliding a wire with a deployable stent at its tip into a blocked blood vessel in the heart. The procedure is done in free-standing surgery centers. Over 99 percent of these procedures go well, but on rare occasions, the wire used to place the stent can rupture the coronary artery, or the balloon used to dilate the hardened artery blows a hole in it. If this happens, emergency open-heart surgery is the only way to save the patient's life. If you're having the procedure done at an ambulatory surgery center with no backup heart surgeon, operating room, or heart-lung bypass machine close by (the equipment required to perform the open-heart operation), you are out of luck.

What's more shocking about heart procedures is that many cardiologists agree that a good number of them don't need to be done. Of the roughly two hundred thousand heart angioplasty procedures done in the United States each year for patients without heart-attack symptoms, 38 percent are done for uncertain indications and 12 percent (or roughly twenty-four thousand) are done for "inappropriate" indications, according to a study published in 2011 in the prestigious *Journal of the American Medical Association* by a forward-thinking group of cardiologists.[11]

A close friend's dad had a heart defibrillator placed and was told it was a routine and safe procedure. At the time, I questioned the need for him to have one put in at all. But I'm not a cardiologist, and I wasn't involved with the family's decision to proceed. So I kept quiet. Unfortunately, he died suddenly during the procedure. This made it especially agonizing for me to read in the 2011 *Journal of the American Medical Association* study that one in five patients who received heart defibrillators didn't meet guidelines to have them placed. In reporting the findings, the *Wall Street Journal* suggested that the overutilization of the $25,000 implantable device was driven by the $4.3 billion market.[12] Medicine is not exempt from the financial incentives of the rest of the world.

Every Specialist Knows

I ask my orthopedic-surgeon friends and colleagues every time I
run into them if it's true that there's too much back surgery going
on. They insist it is true, and it's driven by money. When I ask colleagues in my own field, oncology, about the markup of chemo
drugs and the lack of transparency to patients, they agree it is
prevalent, profitable, and wrong. When I ask cardiologists about
too many stents and devices being put in people, many, though
not all, will agree that some cardiologists are doing too many procedures. My hunch about those who don't is that they're being
discreet out of reluctance to go against their own. Usually, whenever I ask doctors to comment about these matters, I am mightily
impressed by how outraged they are, angry that such things
should go on in their field—a field they are proud of, and want to
be proud of rather than ashamed of. Doctors overall do care about
patients' well-being and are well aware of the perverse incentives
that drive good doctors to do questionable things.

But is it only orthopedics, cancer, and cardiology that overtreat?
As an exercise, I began to ask specialists the question, "What is
the most overutilized thing in your field?"

Pediatricians said, "Antibiotics." Radiologists said, "CAT
scans." Obstetricians said, "C-sections."

All specialists, from allergists to psychiatrists, have at least one
procedure or treatment they complain is overdone. If you ask
around, it appears that *every field* of medicine has one thing that
most people agree they overdo. Each specialist had a story like my
experience with pancreas-cancer treatment. As long as doctors
get paid like sales reps, they're going to sell their service—
whether it's chemotherapy, cardiac stents, or C-sections.

CHAPTER 12

The All-American Robot

TOWERING AT SIX FOOT ELEVEN INCHES tall, like a creature from the movie *Transformers*, it flexes its mechanical arms, each holding a surgical instrument. There's a reason why the manufacturer named it Zeus. As I gaze at the robot working in the operating room next door to mine, I am equally struck by its graceful movements and cold, steely demeanor as it hovers over a patient and performs surgery exactly as I normally do. With sales growing faster than the iPod, this robot is wildly popular in America.[1] As of 2012, it is in every major U.S. hospital and many community hospitals. It's the latest rage. In 2011 alone, this single device performed more than 150,000 routine operations in the United States, up 400 percent from just four years ago.

But what does the robot do better than a human surgeon?

Proponents contend that it's better than a human surgeon because it eliminates resting tremors present with human hands, and it allows for more range of motion with the instruments than with standard handheld instruments (standard laparoscopy). Finally, it can enable surgeons who are not skilled in laparoscopy to now perform it, since complex surgical techniques are easier with the robot than standard laparoscopy. Some doctors who use the robot for heart, oral, and rectal surgery have claimed that it is better for visualization and ease of use.

But my experience gives me a different perspective. The robot is totally controlled by a surgeon, who operates it from a chamber resembling an interactive arcade machine. As a guy who likes to be ahead of the curve, I was eager to give it a try. Strapped to a sophisticated network of sensors detecting my hands' every movement, I felt like an iron man. When my right arm moved, the robot's right arm moved in perfect synchrony as I watched the operation on a screen (even though it was only seven feet away). Instantly I felt immortal, strong, and ready to conquer. It was every Nintendo Wii gamer's dream. The robot does just what you do. It has no mind of its own. It's a giant mimicker—a very expensive pair of remote-controlled human hands. While I have no doubt that robotic surgery technology will improve and may offer superior operations for select procedures, by and large it's not clear that robots currently do the job better than human surgeons.

And these robots cost upward of $2 million a pop—not a small price tag for a health care system that is already straining to save money safely. But our love for new technology often seems to trump financial concerns.

"It's way cool," one fellow surgeon excitedly told me with a giant grin during a training session. But when I asked him if it was worth the huge price tag and thousands of dollars more in disposable parts thrown out after each case, he had no response. Doing some quick math in my head, I calculated that the $140,000 paid for one robot's annual service contract alone could close our hospital's gap in patients' copays and high deductibles and pay for our malpractice-insurance hikes. If only it were that easy.

To learn more, I signed up for a training session. The atmosphere at the training was exceptionally friendly. I was thrilled to learn how to use the new supertoy, as were we all. It was a rare moment of camaraderie. Heart surgeons, gynecologists, urologists, and general surgeons all gathered together in the spirit of a common goal that I hadn't seen since the first year of medical school. After the lecture, we proudly paraded to the training room like suited astronauts walking to the space shuttle on launch day.

We all stood in awe of the new technology, but at no point during our training session did anyone ask, Why are we doing this? Surely the robot must have some benefit, I thought: After all, 70 percent of robots are in community hospitals. Robots were originally developed with several goals in mind, including enabling surgeons to perform surgery in remote locations. But if it were me, I would want my surgeon present in person.

I set out to review all 409 research studies on the robot in the medical literature. In my opinion, none showed any convincing clinical benefit over conventional laparoscopic surgery, except for a few studies the robot company had paid for. One South Korean study that found that robotic surgery had better outcomes concluded that robotic surgery was associated with one less day spent in the hospital. But the researchers themselves had sent the patients home. So this study was not exactly objective. While many studies found a clear benefit to robotic surgery, the comparison group was open surgery, not standard laparoscopic surgery.

Andrew Ibrahim of Case Western Reserve University School of Medicine recently concluded from a comprehensive analysis of America's ten-year experience with robotic surgery that there is not strong evidence to support a benefit to patients.[2] When I get a few beers into my colleagues who promote robotic surgery, they too will often admit that it's mainly a marketing hook to attract patients. Dr. Ibrahim also found numerous studies reporting longer operation times and prolonged setup time while the patient is anesthetized. More alarming, some anesthesiologists have reported that the robot didn't allow them to do emergency CPR during surgery because it got in the way. Some surgeons say the bulky machine also gets in the way when the need arises for an emergency conversion to open surgery to take care of bleeding complications.[3]

But no doctors want to publish their personal experience of deaths from robots that got in the way. Needless to say, those cases don't make it into the published medical literature or the manufacturers' sales pitches.

From my first days of medical school, I remember teachers dazzling the class with impressive technology that could cure disease. Looking to technology for hope is part of the culture of medicine. But in these days when draconian cuts in health care are being considered, we need to judge technology on the basis of outcomes, not on its coolness factor.

As a specialist who treats rare diseases, I recognize that doctors need the freedom to customize patient care, but for far too long now, the payment system we have has rewarded spending more money even if there's no benefit. As a result, expensive gadgets that may have no real clinical benefit can be rapidly adopted. In the case of the surgical robot, it's an arms race. Hospitals are buying them, using them, and marketing them faster than anyone can interpret the scientific data on them. Results of new treatments and operations in medicine should be available to the public in an easy-to-understand way. History shows that we doctors rarely resist the temptation to use new technology—especially if we profit from it.

To know the real story on what's the best care, all you have to do is ask the frontline health care providers. Ask the nurses, surgical technicians, and anesthesiologists who do the robotic-surgery cases what they think. In total, I asked more than one hundred operating room staff, "What's your opinion of robotic surgery?" and unless it was a surgeon who performs robotic surgery, here were the common responses nearly everyone made: "They take forever." "What's the point?" "I hate doing those cases." While some doctors have done so many thousand robotic procedures that their safety profile is as good as that of any other approach, centers with limited experience are at highest risk for mishaps. In studying the subject of robotic surgery, I am convinced that future generations of the robots will yield a superior result for patients for a limited set of procedures. However, looking back over the past "decade of the robot," I wonder how the craze made us spend so many billions of dollars when it resulted in patient outcomes no better than standard minimally invasive surgery.[4]

Medicine isn't the only culture to worship technology over outcomes. As with other industries of highly dedicated professionals, like the military, doctors have their own culture with their own language, values, and internal policing. The United States now owns four times as many surgeon robots as all other countries in the world combined, a fact we should be proud of—*if* it helped patients.[5] Health-policy professors are unanimous that the number-one driver of rising health care costs in the United States is new technology. The surgical robot perfectly symbolizes how our widespread adoption of new, high-tech solutions without proper evaluation of their benefits is breaking the bank.

To examine how the robot industry and hospitals are driving demand, I embarked on a research study on robotic marketing claims made on U.S. hospital websites. I assigned medical student Linda Jin of Washington University School of Medicine to lead the project. Her research uncovered that robotic surgery is being actively marketed on 41 percent of U.S. hospital websites, many of which make unsupported claims of robotic surgery's superiority.[6] Words and phrases like *superhuman* and *improved cancer outcomes* were prevalent, despite the lack of any high-level evidence to support a difference in cancer survival. When hospitals claimed superiority for robotic surgery, they failed to specify the comparison group: Was robotic surgery being measured against traditional open surgery or standard minimally invasive surgery? Curiously, the hospital educational web pages on robotic surgery often did not mention risks, only benefits.

Patients have grown to trust doctors over the centuries, and in the modern era, consumers tend to trust a hospital's website as a source of reliable medical information in a doctor's voice. But they shouldn't. In many cases, hospitals have turned their websites over to device and drug manufacturers that claim to be objective but in fact give the corporate sales pitch. Linda Jin found that one third of U.S. hospitals that promote robotic surgery in their patient-information sections are just using advertising language lifted out of a manufacturer's marketing materials verbatim, without attribution or a company-disclosure statement.

To take a stand regarding the close relationship between device manufacturers and U.S. hospital websites, Johns Hopkins recently announced a ban on industry-authored materials on its official hospital site. Some other hospitals have followed with their own policies.

Drug companies figured out long ago that direct drug-to-consumer marketing works wonders for sales. Bypassing the doctor—by advertising straight to the patient with calculated appeals to buyer psychology, wants, needs, and blind spots—creates demand. Device makers are now taking their cue from the success of drug makers. Robotic surgery is the first example I know of a device manufacturer that has advertised directly to the consumer with gigantic success. In fact, one robot company, Intuitive Surgical, was among the top-performing stocks on the NASDAQ in 2009, in large part from the success of its aggressive advertising campaign.

All of the salesmanship for robotic surgery is working. Patients coming to my office are now asking for it—even demanding it. One patient who needed his appendix removed told me that he wanted the latest state-of-the-art surgery and would do whatever it took to get it. When I told him that I recommended standard laparoscopy to remove his appendix rather than robotic surgery, he left in a huff (even though the robotic surgery would have taken twice as long to do, given the setup time). I wanted to tell him that robotic surgery would mean more time under general anesthesia for him, that it has no patient benefit according to all the top studies, and that it costs the system about $4,000 more per operation. I also wanted to tell him how the *Wall Street Journal* recently reported that after one hospital demonstrated its new robot at a local sporting-event halftime show on live patients, the patients wound up suffering from holes the robot accidentally made in their bladders.[7] I never got to share these points with him. The patient probably had his surgery done robotically by another surgeon, thinking he was getting the better care.

Culture is local. It explains why, in one hospital, some doctors embrace new technology so completely that they get too cozy with industry and become advocates for products, while in another, other doctors tell patients the truth, lay out the data, and partner with their patients to determine the best course of treatment tailored to their goals. Culture explains why some hospitals ban industry marketing from the hospital- and patient-information web content, while other hospitals post industry content without disclosures in order to attract customers with superficial claims. As a society we need to choose which new medical interventions to utilize based on what's best for the patient, not just on coolness. National groups have recently organized to try to make results of medical research available to the public in ways that they can understand and use to make decisions. The new Patient-Centered Outcomes Research Institute is one of those organizations that has a stated mission to help people "make informed health care decisions."[8] But it's not easy. One barrier to access has been the publishing industry. Publishers often charge for online access to research results even though doctors write and review the articles for the publisher for free and publishers generate revenue from drug- and device-company advertisements. In some instances, the prestigious American Medical Association journal charges thirty dollars for online access to research articles funded by taxpayer dollars. A completely taxpayer-funded study my research team conducted on the effectiveness of weight-loss surgery (a study entirely paid for by the federal Agency for Healthcare Research and Quality) was published in a leading medical journal that required that you log in and pay a thirty-dollar fee to access it during the first twelve months the results were available. It doesn't seem fair that you, the consumer, fund research but then must pay an online fee to see the results of it. These barriers symbolize the challenges to making good medical information readily available to patients so they can make informed decisions.

In the case of robotic surgery, what I've learned from the existing body of evidence and my own experience specializing in one of the most complex laparoscopic operations in medicine, the laparoscopic whipple, is that the clinical differences between standard minimally invasive surgery and robotic surgery appear to be very small. Overall, surgeon skill and expertise still trump any potential benefit from the device alone. Thus, for now my advice is to choose a surgeon, not a robot.

PART III

Transparency Time

CHAPTER 13

Drivers of Culture

Mayo

AMONG U.S. MEDICAL CENTERS, none has a better reputation for efficiency and quality than the Mayo Clinic in Rochester, Minnesota. This isn't just an insider's secret; the public is well aware of it, too. People flock from San Francisco, Chicago, and New York—cities with some of the most advanced medical centers in the world—to a remote town an hour-and-a-half drive from the closest international airport. When diplomats, CEOs, and celebrities want to get serious about their care, they often go to Mayo.

Mayo's high level of service and focus on patient-centeredness is the envy of every hospital in America. It has achieved a level of coordination no other hospital has been able to master on a consistent basis—not even Mayo itself, which opened two spin-off hospitals, in Scottsdale, Arizona, and Jacksonville, Florida, that never matched the efficiency of the "mother ship."

During my time at Harvard, Johns Hopkins, and Georgetown, and in my many conversations with colleagues at UCLA, Vanderbilt, and Emory, I've heard the Mayo hospital praised repeatedly. Mayo somehow has been able to coordinate departments that at other hospitals seem to act independent from one another. Nearly every doctor in America has a nightmare story of how this silo organizational approach creates problems resulting from internal competition or a lack of coordination. In fact, medical care in America is littered with stories of mix-ups, delays, and patients falling through the cracks.

This fragmented care frustrates both patients and doctors. If you go to see one doctor, then get referred to another, you might need to wait weeks or months for the second doctor's next available opening. Or a specialist might be able to see you the moment you are referred. You might even be just a few floors away from the specialist, but most medical centers are not set up for walk-ins.

Except at Mayo. At Mayo, you go directly from one doctor's office to another the same day, with a few hours in between—*maximum*. The first doctor can call over to the referring physician and talk to that doctor before he sees the patient who's on the way. This is a doctor's dream come true. I know for a fact that there's nothing more annoying for a doctor than to track down another physician four to six weeks after a referral. Not only is this a huge waste of everyone's time (most of all the patient's), the reality is, when the patient needs to be scheduled for an appointment far into the future, communication between doctors breaks down.

Chris, a busy real estate agent, called my office looking for a doctor to treat his newly diagnosed belly pain. In the era of the Internet and the ever-popular Google search, I now often get this sort of over the transom phone call. With most such inquiries I work hard to call the patient back within twenty-four hours. When I reached Chris, we had a nice chat. I explained to him what probably needed to be done, whom he needed to see in addition to me, and suggested a plan to accommodate his busy schedule. First he needed an examination, then most likely a CAT scan. I told him he also might need to have a colonoscopy that would be performed by another specialist depending on what we found during his initial visit, so he could fly in and out of Baltimore in a short period of time. He was satisfied with my plan and said it resembled what his local hospital had also suggested. Chris was cordial and grateful and thanked me profusely. He informed me, out of courtesy, that he was also talking to doctors' offices at Harvard,

Mayo, and Washington University about possible treatment for his belly pain. Chris was everything I think a modern patient needs to be: an active researcher and strong personal advocate for his own health who took the responsibility to shop around.

Three days later, my secretary followed up to see if he had decided to schedule an appointment at Hopkins. "I'm all set, thank you very much," he replied. To my surprise, we learned that in just those three days, he had traveled to Mayo, been evaluated by an internist and surgeon, had a CAT scan, a colonoscopy, and preoperative preparation tests, and met with an anesthesiologist. On his third day in Minnesota he had colon surgery. He was now in the recovery room. "Wow, *wow*," my secretary and I said to each other in awe. When I had spoken to Chris I felt I'd offered him an expeditious approach to his care. I had to know: What was it about Mayo that allowed them to be so efficient, high quality, and patient-centered?

I wasn't the only one whose curiosity was piqued. Not long ago, the accomplished president of a leading U.S. hospital, in his first year as president, made a pilgrimage to Rochester, Minnesota, with a few close colleagues and staff. They scheduled a day of meetings with Mayo leaders, managers, and accountants, eager to learn the secrets of the Mayo Clinic's efficiency and success.

"Are we all here?" the president asked as his team gathered to walk over to its first appointment that day. The first meeting was in the Gonda Building. Since the hotel was within walking distance of the hospital campus, the members of the delegation arrived on foot, walked into the first building they saw, and sought directions. In the building's lobby, they found a custodian cleaning the floor. "Excuse me, sir. Do you happen to know where the Gonda Building is?" they inquired.

The custodian, a gentleman about sixty years of age, looked up with a smile. "Oh, my," he said. "It's about five blocks from here, and it's a bit confusing."

Without hesitation, he set his cleaning tools down in the corner of the lobby and walked the delegation out of the building, escorting them for five blocks and directly to the Gonda Building's seventh-floor office and the door of their meeting. During the fifteen-minute walk, the custodian peppered them with conversation, getting to know them, asking them where they were from, how their trip was, where they were raised, and how long they were staying in Rochester, among several gestures of hospitality.

"He is ridiculously friendly," one staffer whispered.

The entire group was blown away by the janitor's kindness, generosity, and determination to make sure they got where they were going. Once the delegates arrived at their destination, the janitor then asked to see their itinerary to confirm that they were in fact at the correct office. "Well, it was nice to meet all of you, and have a great visit here at Mayo," he said.

The impressed delegation stood frozen, looking at each other, with everyone thinking the same thing. "Well . . ." the president said, flabbergasted, with a small grin, "we might as well go home now."

The question of what made Mayo great had been answered. Mayo's administrative-system details seemed almost irrelevant. No business formula made Mayo great, nor advertising, nor new technology. It was Mayo's great hospital culture, one that permeated to even the janitorial staff.

Since that visit, many health care experts have gone to Mayo to try to absorb its model. I visited it in 2011. I, too, was blown away. For a surgeon it was like heaven. Every fifty feet in the operating room hallways there was an oasis like I'd never seen before: break rooms stocked with complimentary drinks, tasty sandwiches, and ice cream; a gorgeous room outfitted with plenty of phones to return calls, desk space, computers, televisions, couches to rest on. It was a surgeon's dream come true—a hospital environment that provides ways to get caught up on patient issues while recharging between long, stressful operations. I'd never seen anything like it before in the twenty or so hospitals I had rotated through in my career. What's more, everyone in the hospital seemed to have a spirit, a sense of mission, a feeling that they were all working together to do the right thing. I commented to my host, Dr. Michael Kendrick, "It's almost as if this hospital was designed and run entirely by doctors to make our work day more efficient, comfortable, and productive."

"It was," he replied. He went on to explain how Mayo has stuck to its original principle set forth by the founding Mayo brothers of "providing the best care to every patient through integrated clinical practice."[1] And to do that, they believed in keeping frontline doctors in charge of how the hospital operates.

Culture isn't created overnight. It takes years to establish and it must be nurtured to be sustained, especially in a large health institution. So how does Mayo do it? How did Mayo get my potential patient Chris in and out in such a jiffy, yet with such impeccable attention to detail? On my visit and in my later research I learned some of the fundamental keys to Mayo's success. First, administrators anticipate having to coordinate care. Instead of filling a schedule book with patient after patient, doctors coordinate so that someone in every department is always available for walk-ins. Administrative assistants work hard to coordinate appointments to ensure that a patient's visit is seamless and efficient. It's a true team effort.

When other hospitals try to adopt Mayo's ways of doing things, it often doesn't work. Some health-services researchers say Mayo's standardization of procedures hospitalwide is what makes it unique. Certainly that helps. Administrators there act more like investigative reporters, walking the halls in search of problems to fix.

In my view, Mayo's strong hospital culture of quality, safety, and patient-centeredness is rooted in a strong tradition of listening to employees. This is not something another hospital can just import or start doing overnight, particularly if a hospital has a lot of bad habits to break first. Mayo's culture reminded me of two other hospitals.

Geisinger Medical Center in my hometown of Danville, Pennsylvania, has the same strong tradition of administrators listening to employees and that same spirit of every employee working hard just for a paycheck. Similar to the Cleveland Clinic, the hospital pays its staff on a salary basis, rather than with a strong eat-what-you-kill compensation plan. Geisinger has often been spotlighted nationally for high-quality programs, such as its money-back guarantee that patients won't develop complications after heart surgery. The hospital also leads the country by having the most advanced electronic health record in medicine. Patients communicate with their nurse or doctor by e-mail. The hospital also offers to send patients a copy of tests and records by e-mail, if preferred. The Wi-Fi-enabled medical campus is full of iPad users and patients using online resources.

Mount Auburn Hospital is the smallest and least known of the Harvard-affiliate hospitals. People there care deeply about patient care and safety and will do anything to ensure high-quality care. Its unity of mission humbles the giants of the Harvard hospital system, and the hospital's outcomes are the best I have ever seen. The size of the hospital seems to foster a close relationship between the medical staff and its administrators. Everyone there knows who the administrators are. They all eat together in the same cafeteria. (The Apple computer company follows the same principle, to promote dialogue and flatten the hierarchy.) If Mount Auburn doctors or nurses have a hospital-wide safety concern, it does not require a formal meeting in a detached building with an administrator they've never met before. Management is in touch with the needs and safety concerns of the frontline providers.

If Mayo, Geisinger, and Mount Auburn released results of an employee safety-culture survey at their institutions, they would be at the top. I'd bet that if surveyed, 90 to 99 percent of these hospitals' employees would want to receive their own care there.

Culture

Why do Southwest Airlines crews joke and laugh over the intercom? Why do people at Toyota stop the belt if they have a quality concern? Why do Bostonians pick up trash? And why does a sales associate at the Apple store seem so happy to work there, popping out as soon as you walk into the store, eager to answer any computer question you might have? Culture.

When the U.S. banking and mortgage industries crashed, many blamed it on a culture of greed: Otherwise good people were driven to turn profits using any arguably legal means while turning a blind eye to the potential consequences of their collective actions. When asked how it is able to recruit the most talented programmers in the industry, Google says it's about culture.

In places where the workplace culture is good, results tend to be better. In places where the workplace culture is bad, results can be tragic, like in the division of Morton-Thiokol that manufactured the fatal O-ring that led to the space shuttle *Challenger* explosion. Workers there voiced safety concerns to their higher-ups about the O-ring's inability to withstand temperature changes—but no one was interested in listening.[2] In 1986, the *Challenger* blew up, a national tragedy that might have been avoided had administrators cultivated a culture of open communication for safety concerns with workers.

Similarly, a team of engineers forewarned New Orleans that its levees couldn't weather a major storm. No one listened, and when Hurricane Katrina hit the Gulf Coast, those engineers could only look on in horror as their worst nightmare came true.

One very different culture is Toyota. Toyota executives famously listen, routinely solicit their employees for safety concerns and ideas, and act on them. Known as the Toyota Production Standard, this practice of continuously and formally soliciting staff for their ideas has been touted as a model in the field of quality improvement—a culture of empowering even the lowest-level employees and encouraging them to express their concerns. The Toyota Production Standard is now taught all across academia, including at Harvard Business School and the Johns Hopkins School of Public Health, as a model for quality management. Many other companies and industries have adopted the importance of listening to employees in an effort to improve quality.

A friend of mine, Mike Perry, vice president of a Houston-based subsidiary of AIG, believes that it was a shift in culture that spawned the financial crisis. Married for thirty years with five kids, Mike is known for his leadership, humility, and honesty. His local company, Valic, he told me over the course of an hour one evening, had once been a fun place to work, with a great work ethic, a noble mission, and a high level of job satisfaction—before AIG bought them. Valic kept doing well after the AIG merger, increasing profits by a healthy 8 to 15 percent per year. But each year New York would call to say, We're pleased with your group's increase in profits last year. Can you do it again this year? The Valic execs would reply that they'd try, but of course there were no guarantees. Year after year, the pressure was palpable. It soon became clear that New York didn't care to know any of the details of how they made their 15 percent increase, just so long as they kept it up. Over time, this insistent pressure changed Valic's culture, making its people more stressed, less satisfied, and more worried about being replaced. Increasing gains in profit has inevitable limits for any business. Yet the new culture focused so remorselessly on this metric, it seemed to supplant all other corporate values. As hospitals grow and merge into giant corporations with remote executives, the impact of long-distance management on a hospital culture needs to be kept in check.

A culture can either motivate people to work or to exploit. Enron notoriously created a culture in which management said in more ways than one, We don't care how you make money and we don't want to know. The blind eye is characteristic of a business or organization with a distant management hierarchy—with a resulting culture that penetrates every aspect of the organization.

Culture defines the quality and safety of any community or workplace, and medicine is not exempt. As small hospitals are increasingly becoming large corporate storefronts via the many mergers and acquisitions in health care, it is critical that medicine's culture of putting patients first be preserved, rather than succumb to distant managers. The start to ensuring this community obligation is to measure the teamwork and safety culture and patient outcomes at a local level.

My Near Miss

One typical workday at Johns Hopkins, I walked into the hospital thinking I had a light day. I had four small operations to do, a few patients in the office to see, and a few research meetings. The first two operations went well—ahead of schedule. As I finished meeting with my third patient, I was briskly interrupted by a nurse. One of my patients in the intensive care unit faced a life-threatening complication. I hastened to the ICU to find the problem had been resolved, but I had to spend some time in the unit troubleshooting the case with the resident and a nurse.

Finally I returned to the OR for my third operation of the day. As usual, a new intern was rotating in with me on the operation. I walked into the operating theater to perform a procedure to remove fluid from the lung. The right chest had been nicely scrubbed with Betadine and a window of skin fashioned with sterile towels. Tense with anxiety, the intern asked, "Is this how you like your towels folded?" I smiled at him saying, "It looks good, thanks, buddy." Interns working with a new surgical-faculty member for the first time are often sweating bullets that they don't get perceived early on as incompetent. Relieving their anxiety with an encouraging word often makes them more relaxed.

I was just about to make my incision when the nurse broke the silence in the room.

"Wait. Are we doing the right or left chest? Because it says here left but that looks like the right side."

My heart instantly raced and started beating audibly. I felt as if I were on a battlefield where the fog of war had suddenly pulled back to expose carnage. I looked at the patient, petrified, my scalpel hovering over the chest. It was impossible to tell if the skin window was on the patient's right or left because there were so many towels, drapes, and other equipment on the surgical field.

"Oh, my God. That was close," I said. "Thank you, Linda, for speaking up."

Thanks to the nurse's quick thinking and courage to speak her mind, we were able to adjust the patient's position and perform the surgery on the correct side. (The nervous intern learned a hard lesson about surgical prep, but hopefully also walked away with an important understanding of the need for communication in the OR.) The situation was a classic setup for the kind of mistake that Peter Attia had suffered, with a distraction in the ICU pulling me out of the operating room while the patient was being positioned for surgery. It was a sobering lesson for me. This case was the impetus for creating a surgical checklist.[3]

My near miss wasn't the first time a nurse has prevented a catastrophe for me. My nurses always tell me their safety concerns, and I consider their input invaluable. In a field littered with human error, having nurses and other staff act as a safety net to avoid mistakes makes a huge difference. Creating a culture in which speaking up is encouraged makes a big difference in patient outcomes. Conversely, when staff members don't speak up, safety is compromised.

The Joint Commission on hospital accreditation reports that the vast majority of major medical mishaps result from breakdowns in communication. One young girl at Duke University Hospital got a heart transplant with the wrong blood type, resulting in instant rejection and death.[4] A nurse in the room might have seen that the test for compatibility hadn't been verified and simply asked if the crossmatch had been done. Nurses aren't directly responsible for this, but they know the drill as well as anyone. I'd guess that a nurse might well have noticed here, but just felt too intimidated and low on the totem pole to contradict the all-star team of surgeons in the room. A girl's life might have been saved along with millions of dollars in liability for Duke.

A Culture of Speaking Up

There is one common thread among hospital mishaps: poor communication. Medicine is highly complex, and there are countless ways to make mistakes, large or small. Most can be easily and quickly corrected—when people work as a team and speak out without hesitation. If you ask hospital risk managers what the leading cause of hospital mistakes is, they will tell you they're often the result of someone knowing something wasn't quite right, but not speaking up. The Joint Commission, the accreditation organization for hospitals, reports that breakdowns in communication cause more hospital mishaps than equipment failures and inadequate training combined.

The hospital can be an intimidating place for a health care worker. It has a strong hierarchy. Following orders promptly is valued the same way it is on the battlefield. Defiance is unheard of and punishable with harsh penalties. The nurses and residents taking the orders often don't have as much expertise as the ordering doctors and might question their own knowledge if they are feeling something isn't right. As a trainee at a hospital in the D.C. metropolitan area, I once questioned a doctor's decision to keep a patient on a ventilator. To me, the patient clearly didn't need it and was ready to have the breathing tube removed. Saying so lit the doctor up. His eyes opened wide and his face glistened with sweat as he scrambled for words. He retorted huffily, "What do you know about ventilators? I've been doing this for ten years!" The next day, a Saturday, his senior partner was covering for him and agreed with me that the patient should have been taken off. But my exchange with the first doctor taught me another tough lesson about the dangers of speaking out.

It's worse the lower down the hierarchy you go. Nurses often have safety concerns. Whether they feel free to voice those concerns depends on hospital culture. I readily admit that nurses have saved my butt dozens of times, especially when I was a trainee. I've misread lab results, forgotten to check chest X-ray reports, and even walked into the wrong patient's room. All these mistakes were immediately caught by nurses who felt comfortable correcting me. Among the nurses, I have a reputation for being soft-spoken, kind, and unflappable.

Conversely, one of my coresidents had a reputation for being a loose cannon—easily angered and known to swirl around like a Tasmanian devil when provoked. Nurses would routinely say how much they hated working with him. Some mornings, I'd walk onto the hospital ward and witness the carnage of his overnight temper tantrums—nurses slumped over on chairs looking as if they had just come out of a boxing ring. Many were humiliated by his yelling and demeaning comments. As a result, the nurses and staff called him less often with patient updates. And when he made mistakes like I did, they were less likely to help him out. A few times, nurses with serious safety concerns would call me at home on nights I wasn't on duty to share their concerns. When I would ask if they called my coresident, they'd often say they'd tried but he'd brushed them off, acting annoyed. Patients under his care suffered because of these communication breakdowns. All this renegade needed was someone higher up the food chain—somebody with authority over his career—to take him aside and tell him to correct his attitude toward his coworkers. That never happened. He continued to terrorize his staff to the detriment of his patients.

To prevent mistakes, the hospital culture must permit free speech. To my students at Johns Hopkins, I teach that yelling at a nurse even once can intimidate them so that they fear you, harming communication and posing a danger to patients. This intimidation can last for years.

At one point I happened to notice that needlestick injuries were shockingly common in the operating room, and that trainees or nurses often didn't speak up when they get stuck. To me they were a marker of the culture. If they were fearful about speaking up about their own injuries, then it seemed to me that they were also unlikely to speak up about patient-safety concerns. I later conducted a research study of needlesticks as a proxy for uncommunicative medical culture, together with Ali Al-Atar, an MD/Ph.D.–combined degree student at the time. We surveyed interns and residents at fifteen academic medical centers, asking anonymous interviewees how often they spoke up about a needlestick injury. To our amazement, we found that about half didn't do or say anything. The study appeared in the *New England Journal of Medicine*, confirming what Ali and I had observed throughout our training: Employees don't speak up enough.[5]

How does a hospital create a culture of speaking up? Dr. Bryan Sexton, whom I mentioned in chapter two, developed this metric: "I feel comfortable speaking up when I sense a patient safety concern: agree/disagree" for the safety-culture survey that was administered to sixty U.S. hospitals. Here's what we found when we surveyed hospital employees:

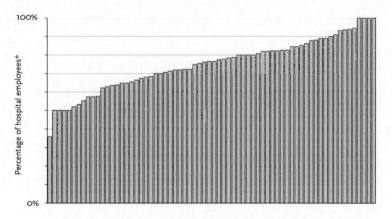

Each bar corresponds to one hospital

*Employees per hospital who feel comfortable speaking up when sensing a patient safety concern

The response varied by hospital. At some, hardly any of the workers felt comfortable speaking out when they saw a safety concern. At other hospitals, nearly everybody did. These results tracked with other objective measures of hospital performance.

I have written more than one hundred original scientific articles in my academic career. You can never predict which will make a real contribution to medical science and which won't. One study that I thought would be the least significant wound up my most-cited paper—a study Drs. Bryan Sexton, Peter Pronovost, and I did that broke down teamwork scores by type of hospital employee (doctor versus nurse versus anesthesia provider versus surgery technician) as revealed by our survey. We asked each type of provider to rate their colleagues on the quality of their teamwork on a scale from 0 to 100, with 100 representing a perfect score. To our surprise, here's what we found:

All participants rated teamwork among their own kind very well: Doctors work well with other doctors and nurses with other nurses. In addition, doctors rated their teamwork with the nurses as very good (88 percent). But the results from nurses rating doctors

Caregiver position being rated

		Surgeon	Anesthesiologist	Nurse	CRNA
	Surgeon	85	84	88	87
	Anesthesiologist	70	**96**	89	92
	Nurse	**48**	63	81	68
	CRNA	58	75	76	93

Caregiver position performing rating (left vertical axis label)

Teamwork score (0–100) by caregiver type (CRNA stands for Certified Registered Nurse Anesthetists)

showed a big gap in perception. Nurses rated their teamwork with doctors as bad (48 percent), contradicting communication doctors reported as great. This was a humbling result, indicating that doctors need to be more self-aware. Surgeons may master technical skills, but this study says we have not mastered nontechnical skills as well as we might think.[6]

This disconnect would never have surfaced without an anonymous survey. With this in mind, Dr. Sexton and I conducted field observations of clinical interactions at my hospital. He pointed out something I'd never really noticed before: The staff didn't know the names of the other people they were working with in the operating room. Students, residents, nurses, and anesthesiologists would come and go freely, depending on their shift schedules. When I thought about it, I realized I knew this to be true from my own experience. I might work with as many as thirty other health care workers, yet at best I knew the names of only a few of them. How could we ask people to create a culture of communication when they were working in almost complete anonymity? How could there be accountability and congeniality when no one knew something as basic as their colleagues' names?

When two drivers who come to a four-way stop try to cut each other off, they can fly off the handle at each other. But if a bystander, recognizing them, calls out, "Hey, that's my son's teacher" about one driver and "Hey, that's my dad's friend" about the other, the drivers stop and apologize. What happened? Why did the recognition make them act civil? When the other driver became a real person and was no longer anonymous, people felt compelled to act with civility.[7] Anonymity fosters incivility.

We formed a focus group. The nurses echoed that they felt more comfortable speaking up when they were known by name. In addition, they said being ordered to do something by someone who didn't know their name was insulting. Being called by name restored their dignity, they said.

After asking operating-room members whether they felt comfortable speaking up, we decided to implement briefings before surgery in which the team members ran down a short, surgical checklist easy enough to complete in a few minutes. A key element of the checklist was team introductions. After implementing the checklist for twelve weeks in a trial group, we resurveyed the participants. The nurses, technicians, and anesthesia providers reported feeling dramatically more comfortable speaking up after briefings prior to surgery in which they had all been introduced to their team. They also had better teamwork scores.[8] Teams reported better awareness of the patient's name, the correct procedure, and the side of the patient that the procedure was to be performed on. We concluded that major errors such as operating on the wrong patient, conducting the wrong procedure, or operating in the wrong place could be better prevented if a speaking-up culture was encouraged by presurgery briefings. Surgeons sometimes complain that the checklist will take up valuable time—but we found that the briefings in fact led to fewer delays in the operating room because they gave the team a chance to anticipate and discuss any problems that might emerge.

In 2006, I was honored to be invited by the World Health Organization (WHO) to be part of a small group of doctors charged with the task of improving surgical safety worldwide. A dozen of us gave presentations with "pitches" for the project. Mine discussed the local success of our checklist program at Johns Hopkins, including our research findings that the checklist increased compliance with evidence-based practices and enhanced the safety culture in the operating room.[9] My pitch was selected and we began a year-long process of expanding our surgical checklist into an official WHO document to be applied to every type of medical procedure in every country in the world. Drs. Atul Gawande, Alexander Haynes, Bill Berry, Tom Weiser, and others led the effort, and later did a research study on the implementation of the WHO checklist. They found that it reduced some complications dramatically and raised the level of safety in the OR.[10] Gawande's book *The Checklist Manifesto* brilliantly explains the value of checklists for mastering complex procedures, not just in medicine, and shows how, in a medical setting, this simple intervention can save lives.

Progress in the United States toward adopting briefings and checklists has been highly variable. As with the adoption of minimally invasive surgery, some doctors simply don't like to do them, so they don't, despite clear evidence in the medical literature that they are better for patients. Many doctors here thanked me for the innovation, but others detest the idea. Various initiatives are ongoing to engage doctors and nurses to use checklists to improve hospital culture and patient safety. You might ask if your hospital uses them before your next surgical procedure.

In talking about these issues nationwide, I am struck by the high percentage of doctors who express the same frustrations at how we've strayed as a profession from the ideals that drew us to medicine. Doctors are now speaking out on these topics and are hungry for ways to improve medicine's culture. Partnering with the American College of Surgeons, Dr. Peter Pronovost and I are now leading an $8 million grant-funded project to create specialty-specific small groups at hospitals to improve hospital culture. The small-group forums, called CUSP (Comprehensive Unit-Based Safety Program) groups, bring together doctors in a given specialty, the nurses they work with, and hospital executives to discuss local safety concerns.[11] Such programs have been shown in new studies to result in improved patient outcomes and to help restore medicine to its original values.[12] Doctors are eager for common-sense solutions to fix our disjointed health care system.

CHAPTER 14

Healthonomics

CHECKLISTS AND MEDICAL-UNIT group meetings with administrators are a few common-sense solutions that are quickly gaining attention in health care. But there are many other innovations that hospitals can adopt that, in my opinion, can have an even larger impact on modern medicine. These interventions are simple and can make your personal medical care better and safer through increased transparency.

Open Notes

Sue, a pleasant young accountant, came to my office complaining of abdominal pain. She wasn't sure what was causing it, but had a few ideas. "Could this be from my Bikram yoga?" "Did my late-night ice cream cause the pain?" "Does having unprotected sex have anything to do with it?" were some of the theories she tested out on me. After getting her story down and examining her, I discussed a few things she could try and suggested that she have some lab tests done. Throughout our visit, I took notes. When we were through with the visit, she looked down at my notes with a bit of suspicion. I paused and looked at her in case she had a departing question.

"What did you write about me?" she asked politely, but with a whiff of distrust.

I decided to probe her question a bit. I learned she was concerned that I thought she was either nuts or an ice cream addict. She thought a false representation of her might follow her in her permanent medical record and was worried that she was doing a poor job communicating her pain to me. In the course of our dialogue, I also learned that she wasn't quite sure why I was recommending an ultrasound, although I thought I had told her.

Have you ever left a doctor's office feeling as though you weren't on the same page as the doctor? Patient-satisfaction studies show that many people don't feel totally satisfied. Some can't remember the name of their diagnosis, or how to spell it, or their treatment plan—or they forget parts. Some wonder if the doctor has really heard and understands them. I sometimes learn after questioning a patient that some don't feel they are being heard at all. Or, after they tell their story, they want to edit it, after having had the time to think about it: "Actually, my pain isn't so much in the stomach area, it's really in the lower chest; and it tends to come and go after meals." Days or weeks after seeing a patient in my office, I'll sometimes get a call asking, "Doctor, can you tell me again when I should take the medication?" or, "Doctor, can you tell me again if you want me to get the CAT scan?"

Most doctors' offices are used to answering a stream of follow-up questions from patients who need something clarified after a visit. Some offices have devised creative ways to filter these calls to deal with the high volume, the way your cable TV company does. Yet what we doctors hear about can be just the tip of the iceberg. There is certainly a lot more confusion out there than we know. Research shows that half of all patients don't comply with the treatment regimen their doctor outlines, so confusion is clearly rampant. This is not necessarily the patient's—or the doctor's— fault. Many of my patients are so anxious about hearing bad news, they aren't listening very well to what I'm saying except for the verdict: you do or don't have cancer, or you do or don't need surgery. Listening so hard for the bottom line can mean not hearing other things I say during their visit. Sometimes patients just get overwhelmed. For this reason, patient-advocacy groups recommend that patients bring a friend or family member with them for important doctor visits so there is a second set of ears to listen while the patient is absorbing what could be a life-changing diagnosis.

We doctors also get overwhelmed, but in a different way. Seeing twenty to thirty patients in a single clinic day, I might be juggling dozens of cases at once involving hundreds of medical issues. On busy days, cases can start to blur together. Once, one of my residents interrupted me to tell me about a patient I saw the previous week who had just showed up in the ER with recurrent belly pain.

"Is this the guy who had a part of his colon removed in the past?" I asked.

"Yes, I'm pretty sure he did," the resident told me. Of course, we do confirm everything, but we are also human. The medical histories of hundreds of patients in a single week can sometimes get confused.

To have more accurate notes, I decided to open them up to patients by dictating my notes with them listening in at the end of their visit. I say, "I'm going to take a minute to dictate my notes into the record. Will you please interrupt me and correct me if you hear something that I missed or doesn't seem right to you?" Every patient has gladly told me to go right ahead.

"I also have high blood pressure," was a correction one older patient blurted out. Another said, "My prior surgery was actually on the right, not the left side." Another patient interrupted me midsentence and said, "No, I said I take twenty milligrams, not twenty-five milligrams, of Lipitor." When patients correct me, I thank them and then dictate into the record, "Correction," and add the updated information.

Transparency builds trust. Being able to review your doctor's notes in writing might be even better, particularly if you could add your own comments, perhaps via the web. Transparency plus collaboration puts patient and doctor literally on the same page, so people no longer have to wonder what their doctor is thinking or whether it radically diverges from what they understand.

As many as half of all medical records have been shown to contain mistakes in medication lists and other key elements of background information.[1] With open notes, blatant errors in a person's medical record could be proofed.[2] Personally, I would love to get the patient's feedback and corrections, or side notes, even after-thoughts like "I don't think I have a flu, but my boyfriend in-sisted I get this checked out" or "I also remember now that I had appendicitis when I was a kid." A brief message like this would allow the doctor to gauge what the patient is thinking while add-ing a check layer for transcription errors. It would also be thera-peutic, empowering patients to feel they are a part of their own care—an important principle for the treatment of many illnesses. And it would help just to remind patients of information they need to know, in case they forget.

Harvard doctor-researchers Jan Walker and Tom Delbanco are trying out "open notes" at Harvard and Beth Israel hospitals in Boston, and my hometown hospital, Geisinger Medical Cen-ter, has begun giving patients online access to their doctors' notes. So far, both patients and doctors love it. Dr. Delbanco be-lieves that it is the traditional system of secrecy that violates the trust and duties of the doctor-to-patient relationship. He main-tains that patients have a right to their medical information, and transparency will produce better medicine and safer care. Open notes would cure patient worries and hidden sources of error in medical records. While the program is in its pilot stage, and the special issues of psychiatric diagnoses need to be worked out, or excluded, open notes represents a new level of transparency in medicine. I predict that efforts such as open notes will increase the honesty of the doctor-patient relationship and make it work better.

Family–Centered Care

When my brother was in the emergency room with an orthopedic issue, I went to the hospital to visit him. Even though I used to work at the same hospital, being a visitor I experienced the place in a completely different way than what I was used to. No one cared that I was a surgeon; to them I was just another visitor. I really caught a glimpse of what life is like on the other side of the system. Talk about feeling unwelcome—it was rough. I was told sternly that the strict visiting-hour rules meant I had to be out by eight o'clock P.M. I didn't have access to the hospital cafeteria after six-thirty P.M., so there was nowhere to eat. My questions were answered with an evasiveness I knew all too well.

Having worked at a neighboring hospital in the same city where, more than once, I discovered a dead patient in the bathroom or hallway, I wanted to stay close to my brother at night. I knew how nurses could get overloaded and spread thin. With my brother's condition, I felt he required more attention than what the nurse on duty could provide. My request to spend the night with him, however, was denied. I politely inquired a few times about making an exception. Each time I was treated as though I were some kid or deviant who would be accommodated to any degree only with extreme reluctance. The second night, I finally wore them down and spent the night in a hard wooden chair without being offered any pillows or blankets. The next day, when the doctors met to discuss my brother, they said little to me. As the doctors never said when they would be back to check on my brother, it was nearly impossible to plan being in my brother's room when they were. There was no collaboration or communication. In short, I felt as if a wall existed between them and us.

The patient's family is a critical component of the patient's care team. Recognizing this, leaders at Johns Hopkins have decided to try something radical. Declaring all visiting hours open, Lisa Rowen, director of surgical nursing at the time, established an open-visitation policy, including encouraging one designated member of the family to spend the night in the patient's room. A comfortable sleeping area with pillows and blankets in each room has been set up. Family members are educated as to what warning signs to watch for in their loved one's recovery and how to report any concerns to the staff. In addition, a designated family member is invited to join the doctors and nurses for rounds in which they discuss the patient's plan for the day. There are a few rules: Conversation must be civil, and the family member might be asked to step away over certain sensitive issues (such as mental-illness or addiction concerns). The family member is given time to ask questions at the end. In addition, in order to encourage family involvement, a family lounge has been set up on each floor with a computer and Internet, a phone, a microwave, and a small kitchen stocked with food. Rather than just reluctantly *accommodating* family by bending archaic rules, the hospital ended the age-old divide by *welcoming* families to the care team.

It all made so much sense—and patients' families love it. We call the new program Family-Centered Care. Recently I was proudly explaining how it works in a speech I was giving in East Africa. The doctors in the audience started to chuckle. I stopped and asked them if they had heard of our new program before.

"We've been doing it that way for centuries," a senior surgeon from Tanzania responded from the audience. "You Americans are just now figuring it out," he added with a giant grin.

About six months later, one of my patients who lived in Latin America told me that being able to have his family in the room at all times caring for him was a refreshing reminder of life when he was hospitalized in his home country. He explained that in most of the developing world in which he traveled, families stay in the hospital room and are in charge of much of the nursing care, such as feeding the patient and changing dressings under the doctor's orders. In fact, most docs I know overseas say they've been doing it this way for years, and they find it amusing that we are only now discovering their ancient idea.

Family presence is particularly helpful in reducing one of the nation's leading in-hospital mishaps: falls. Falls by weak and disoriented patients injure and even kill thousands of patients each year—so much so that the Joint Commission and the Institute for Healthcare Improvement require falls to be reported annually and hold conferences to address the problem. The National Quality Forum, the nation's largest medical-quality group, prioritizes fall prevention as its number-two patient-safety goal for America, second only to reducing infection rates. I'm convinced that the common-sense policy to encourage a family member to stay in the room may have saved more lives than the newer cancer drugs last year.

High Fives

Obtaining informed consent from patients on the hospital wards was a task often relegated to interns and trainees. To get the patient's consent, someone has to discuss the operation and all its risks with them. One day there was a patient who needed a major heart operation. I walked in and did my best to explain the risks and indications (even though I had seen only a few patients undergo the operation myself). Armed with my textbook knowledge of the heart operation, I began to explain the procedure to the patient, then asked him to sign the consent form.

"What's the recovery like?" he inquired. I told him that most patients stay in the hospital for about a week after surgery.

"No, I mean, what's the recovery *like*?" he persisted. I repeated to him that he would be in the hospital for about a week and that he would likely start eating and walking on day two after his surgery.

"No, you're not hearing me," he said. "*What's* the recovery like?" I finally realized he meant the recovery at home, i.e., getting around, being in pain, and so on. Truth was, I didn't know—I'd never seen anyone recover at home from an operation. In fact, I'd never even seen anyone in a follow-up office visit after a heart operation. Needless to say, he wasn't satisfied with my lack of knowledge about what to expect, and concluded that he didn't want the surgery.

"I had a good life. I'd rather just go home and be."

My mind raced to my own reality. It was well-known among interns that if an attending senior surgeon found out that a patient refused surgery close to surgery date, duck for cover. Mine would surely be livid—angry that I'd lost a case. I'd suffered this surgeon's rage before and didn't want to experience it again. Especially since I'd been up for thirty hours nonstop and was exhausted, both physically and emotionally.

I explained the situation to my upper resident. As a favor to me, he offered to rescue the situation. He went into the room and was in there for twenty minutes with the door shut. Knowing this resident, I'm sure he sugarcoated the complications and gave the patient a promising picture of the recovery. My friend emerged with an angry look on his face. "We're in deep trouble," he told me. "He won't have it done."

We figured the chief resident would be our last chance before we had to tell the attending surgeon. He rushed down between operations. After an eight-second briefing, he ran into the room and closed the door. Twenty minutes later, he emerged like a shuttle reentering the atmosphere. "He signed," he said, smiling and raising his hand for a high five. The team all high-fived him back, glad that the wrath of the attending surgeon would be averted.

That year, I witnessed hundreds of similar situations in which explaining a complex procedure was framed as how to get the job done: I was asked to help get people to possibly sign their life away, to obtain their informed consent even when I was hardly well-informed about their case myself. I watched the senior surgeons explain a procedure while understating the potential for complications, sometimes giving a skewed picture of the risks and long-term consequences. Instead, things were framed with John Wayne–style bravado: "We're going to go after it and get it out."

Marshall Baker, one of my coresidents, and I made a pact that we would find a way to be more honest with patients when we got to be attending surgeons. We tried to think of exactly how, but couldn't decide. Then one day in my first year as an attending surgeon on the faculty at Johns Hopkins, a patient asked me that same question: What's the recovery like? I gave her all the stats and promised that I'd be available to her throughout her recovery. Again, there was a disconnect between us. She wanted to hear something she could understand, something that wasn't so abstract.

It happened that I had a patient in the next room in for a follow-up visit for the same type of operation, so I thought, why don't they talk? I walked next door and asked my recovering patient if she would be willing to talk to someone thinking of having the same surgery. She jumped at the opportunity. For about fifteen minutes they chatted and I came in for the last five minutes of their conversation. The challenges of the recovery were out there. My new patient was now comforted by being able to see and talk to a recovering patient.

I now ask all of my patients if they would be willing to help out other patients considering having the same surgery, regardless of whether their recovery was smooth or prolonged. Now my patients can call a few past patients and get peace of mind before going under the knife. They get the real story on how long it takes before they can cook a meal or mow the lawn again directly from the source. Moreover, patients feel better going into surgery when the result is tangible and less theoretical. While doctors have faith in statistics and love sharing our opinions, I realized patients value personal experience from someone who's been in their shoes as much as they do my expert perspective.

As a doctor, I prefer a mutual decision to simply telling somebody what to do. Of course, I weigh in with my recommendation. And for some patients, less is more. Some ask me not to tell them the statistics on who does well and who doesn't. Many cancer patients just tell me to take the darn thing out no matter what the risks, costs, or complications. But increasingly in an era when consumers are learning to research online, patients are ready for dialogue with their physicians. I was trained ten years ago in an era of "You're forty, it's time for your mammogram," but a new generation of doctors and patients wants the conversation to go more like, "You're forty now, and the American Cancer Society recommends starting having annual mammograms, but here are the pros and cons of starting now as opposed to some time later."

Similarly, for men, instead of blindly recommending a prostate-specific antigen test (PSA) at age fifty, doctors are discussing the controversy over this recommendation by telling people that an annual PSA test is what the American Cancer Society recommends, while outlining the risks and benefits. Perhaps Google has done more than any hospital initiative to make medicine more transparent. Thanks to Google, patients can easily be well-read on medical recommendations and their controversies. Often they just want a respected partner to share in their decision-making process.

Shared Decision Making: A New Model for Medical Care

Doctors who do procedures are known to understate their complications. We want to reassure our patients and sometimes we fear
scaring them off. The same confidence that allows us to do our job
well can also skew our perspective (though sometimes you want a
cocky surgeon). Self-confident practitioners like to get to work. The
complication rates a doctor will quote out of textbooks and the
medical literature, however, are generally two to three times higher
in the real world. This is a well-known bias in the literature that
in the medical community is called publication bias. It refers to
the fact that only doctors with low complication rates dare submit
their results to a medical journal; thus, the rates reflected in the
scholarly literature are all much lower than the national average.[3]
My research team found, for example, that even though patients
are often quoted a pancreas-surgery mortality rate of 1 percent
based on published studies, the real-world mortality rate is closer
to 7 percent.

After I started letting new patients talk to other patients about
their outcomes, I learned that many other doctors were doing
something similar, using videotapes and pamphlets prior to a procedure to spell out potential real-world complications in lay terms
for patients, using national averages. Spelling out all the possibili-
ties allowed the patients to become well-informed before deciding
to proceed.

The instructional pamphlets and videos are part of a larger effort to have doctors and patients talk honestly and reach a real
agreement about treatment, rather than expecting the patient to
just obey doctor's orders. The movement is called shared decision
making. Popularized by doctors at Dartmouth and McMaster
University medical schools and championed by doctors' organizations and individual practices, shared decision making is being
adopted by many doctors' offices today.[4]

Michael Barry is a past president of the prestigious Society of
General Internal Medicine and a champion of the shared decision-
making model of care, which he uses routinely in his practice at
Massachusetts General Hospital. Knowing that patients aren't

always fond of statistics and percentages of risks, he walks them through the materials and gives them his best advice. Every now and then a patient will, after being given the time to digest these materials, decide against moving forward with a particular test or therapy.

Drs. Albert Mulley and John Wennberg of Dartmouth are so enthusiastic about this approach they've founded a rapidly growing organization called the Informed Medical Decisions Foundation (informedmedicaldecisions.org), which provides tools for doctors' offices, funds demonstration sites, and hopes to take its model to other countries around the world as well. They have initiatives at the University of North Carolina at Chapel Hill, the Oregon Rural Practice-based Research Network, and the University of California, San Diego. Everyone I talked to who has participated in the program loves it and speaks of its intellectual honesty, its transparency, and its empowerment of patients to make decisions with the guidance of a physician.

CHAPTER 15

Candid Cameras

HOW CAN WE ENSURE ACCOUNTABILITY across the field of health care? In principle, most doctors and most hospital administrators agree that accountability is a good thing. But when it comes to being accountable themselves, they are often less enthusiastic. This is only human nature. Taking the extra effort to follow procedures meticulously or keep records of our performance can seem burdensome. And reducing your own accountability can protect your reputation and cover up sins. You are freer to do what you want without having to bother about how other people will react. But a lack of accountability can alienate those you serve and fuel distrust. Moreover, knowing you *are* accountable improves your performance.

A powerful tool in the quest for accountability is the camera. We have seen its value in many fields beyond medicine. The instant replay in sports now settles disputed calls, and security cameras help make a walkway safer. In the field of law enforcement, video cameras can hold both citizens and police accountable. If a few people complain to a city police department about an officer's behavior, typically nothing will happen. But cell phone videos taken by bystanders can capture rogue police officers abusing their authority, and vehicle cameras are now on police cars to record civilian-police interactions.

Educating and encouraging doctors to comply with evidence-based practices is a struggle as old as the problem of getting automobile drivers to comply with the speed limit. But one innovation in the field of motor-vehicle safety has dramatically increased compliance with safety laws overnight—cameras. For a century, educational efforts and radio advertisements begging drivers to be compliant with the law were notoriously low yield. Today, prominent cameras on the side of a road hold drivers accountable for their driving, and cameras at intersections send a strong message to drivers who think of running a red light. These interventions work. Where cameras are in use, compliance with traffic laws has risen and been sustained.[1]

Cameras for Quality

Modern medicine's general lack of accountability is a problem that doesn't just annoy patients. It has long bothered many doctors who are at the top of their field, like Dr. Doug Rex—the most famous name in gastroenterology (GI) worldwide. As past president of the largest GI doctors' association, he has had many landmark accomplishments in medicine, such as putting colon-cancer screening on the map and creating standardized guidelines on how to perform a proper colonoscopy. Because of Dr. Rex's leadership and seminal research, everyone in America is told to have a colonoscopy every five to ten years starting at age fifty to look for colon cancer and suspicious precancerous polyps. To date, Dr. Rex continues to be the best-known and busiest "endoscopist" in the United States for complex polyps and has made his hospital (Indiana University Health) the highest-volume endoscopy center in the country. He has trained thousands of GI doctors and is known by his trainees simply as the godfather. I have talked to some of his former students and they describe him the same way—dedicated, confident, and meticulous. If ever there were an icon in the field of GI medicine, it would be Dr. Rex.

Dr. Rex has been deeply bothered by the widespread sloppiness of doctors in performing colonoscopies in America. He maintains that many doctors in his own field rush through colonoscopies, taking little time to inspect the colon carefully. As a result, many cancers and precancerous polyps are missed, and manifest years later at later stages.

"There are a lot of bad colonoscopies done out there," Dr. Rex explains.[2]

A thorough colonoscopy requires meticulous scrutiny of every nook and cranny of the colon. It takes time. It takes attention to detail. For years, Dr. Rex and other experts in his field have published articles showing that detection rates range widely by doctor. According to Dr. Rex, the quality of the procedure varies dramatically, even at the nation's most reputable hospitals and those listed as "the best" in popular magazines.

"It comes down to the doctor's attitude," Dr. Rex concludes. In the same way that people have different personality types, some doctors are obsessive-compulsive by nature and others are risk takers. Some are even more fatalistic by nature. But when you're dealing with another person's life, doctors should not be taking risks, he adds.

For many years, Dr. Rex was frustrated that he could not study the widespread colonoscopy-quality problem because he knew that a doctor's procedure note in the patient's chart is often curt, sloppy, and in no way captures the thoroughness of the procedure. Based on colonoscopies he repeated (from patients referred by other doctors), Dr. Rex had seen firsthand that some doctors miss critical cancers and polyps.

Dr. Rex had a strong suspicion that even some colonoscopies performed within his own famed center were substandard. To evaluate the quality or thoroughness of the procedure as it was being done by seven of his partners, he secretly began to watch videos of their procedures stored in the system in the procedure area. As he watched the videos, he was shocked at how the length and the quality of the procedure varied dramatically at his own top center. Blinded to the name of the partner that did the procedure, he and his research team began to formally record the amount of time that each doctor spent looking for tumors. He also assigned a quality score based on how well the doctor inspected suspicious-looking areas. After watching one hundred procedures and recording this information, he announced to his seven partners that he would be timing and scoring the videos of their future procedures (even though he was already doing it). Overnight, things changed radically. All of a sudden, the average length of the procedures done by his partners increased by 50 percent and the quality score increased by 30 percent.[3] Same doctors, same hospital, same doctor pay, same patient bills. The only thing different was that the doctors knew that somebody was going to be watching the video of what they were doing.

Seeing the dramatic effect accountability added to patient care, Dr. Rex went a step further. He asked his next 250 patients if they wanted a copy of the video of their procedure. Overwhelmingly, 81 percent said yes.[4] An impressive percentage, considering some patients are geriatric and are not computer savvy. Using a formal questionnaire, Dr. Rex then asked patients who wanted their video why they wanted it. The leading answer was for "review" followed by "to have better records." Most striking, 64 percent of respondents said they were willing to pay to get a video copy of their procedure, a strong affirmation that patients want more transparency in their medical care.

A sampling of procedure videos should be reviewed externally by peers and examined when complications occur. Yet such peer review of procedure videos remains a rarity in modern medicine, in part because these videos are seldom recorded and in part because there is no mechanism or impetus to perform such peer review.

In the current era of medicine, many procedures now employ video—but the record button is either switched off or the video is deleted when the next procedure records over it. To see if my patients would want a copy of their videoed procedure, I began offering them a copy. Their response was enthusiastic. Now when I perform a laparoscopic operation, I download the video that is displayed on the operating-room TV monitor from the camera at the tip of the laparoscopic instrument and give it to patients afterward on a thumb drive. Some like to watch it. Some show it to their referring doctor. And some smartly upload it to their private electronic health record in the cloud like HealthVault.com or Dossia.org.

Just ten years ago, this would have been almost impossible, since videos from the procedure area required a blank VHS tape. Recorded video of medical procedures has broad quality-improvement implications. The cardiologist in Baltimore who put in more than five hundred unnecessary heart stents likely would have been caught earlier if each of his patients had a copy of their angiogram video X-ray showing that their artery was not blocked enough to warrant a stent.

What Dr. Rex's studies taught the medical community is that the same principle that city governments learned with newly installed traffic cameras applies to medicine. When someone is watching, compliance with guidelines radically improves. Making video records available to patients and their doctors is a real game changer and, I believe, can strengthen the patient-doctor trust.

There are other ways cameras can improve medical care. In an era when 93 percent of nurses and 43 percent of physicians report having recently witnessed disruptive behavior, when hand-washing compliance remains highly variable, and when many doctors still do not use preprocedure checklists despite their established benefit, video is an invaluable tool to promote good behavior and compliance with best practices.[5]

Even after the WHO declaration that hand washing decreases hospital-acquired infections and saves lives, compliance in hospitals remains a major struggle. Most hospitals have compliance rates around 40 percent, if they even keep track of it. At Johns Hopkins, each week I receive a report on how we are doing—we use unidentified observers, so-called secret shoppers—to spot-check hand-washing compliance. But secret shoppers can be inaccurate at reporting, maybe because they're not always secret. At Long Island's North Shore University Hospital, roaming secret shoppers were reporting that 60 percent of staffers entering a room had washed their hands. But the hospital went a step further and installed cameras at washing areas. They found a dismal 6.5 percent rate of hand washing. The most striking and important result of the North Shore initiative was that the cameras had a powerful effect. With staffers getting feedback from the cameras, compliance rates rose to over 90 percent and stayed there.[6]

At Vanderbilt, Dr. Matt Weinger and Dr. Michael Higgins have installed cameras throughout their hospital and are studying the data. Surgeons give it mixed reviews, but, tellingly, videotaping gets 100 percent enthusiastic support from nurses. In 2007, brain surgeons at Brown University's hospital, the largest university medical center in Rhode Island, were fined for operating on the wrong side of the brain on three patients. Five wrong-side surgeries were reported over the next two years, two by the same doctor.[7] The state fined the hospital $150,000 and mandated installation of video cameras in all operating rooms. The hospital now has cameras, but no consensus on what to do with its video data. Hospital lawyers hate it; yet increasingly, some doctors are supporting it.

The average American has 9.2 procedures in a lifetime, according to the latest studies by Dr. Atul Gawande.[8] As a surgeon, I know I'd love to be able to see videos of key past operations before I "go in." Like a pro athlete reviewing video of his last game, leaving the hospital with a flash drive with a video of my procedure would only help improve my future procedures. On camera, people behave better, just as people drive better when they know they're passing a videotaped speed trap. Adherence to evidence-based protocols such as surgical checklists would probably also improve. (The current compliance rate is around 40 percent.)[9] In the same way that a cockpit flight recorder serves as a check on professionalism and protocol compliance, so too would videotaping improve professionalism and communication in the operating room.

Traditional medical records are notoriously scant, filled with nonstandardized notations written by a doctor, such as "colonoscopy negative." Dr. Rex's simple study at his hospital introduced a powerful new concept in medicine. If applied widely, videotaping has the potential to transform medicine by adding accountability to an otherwise poorly documented and poorly monitored health care system. I'm convinced that in the future, patients' medical records will routinely include video of their key procedures, without which their records will seem archaic. Imagine a neurosurgeon who calls up a radiologist about a brain tumor on an MRI scan being told by the radiologist that he can only see the radiologist's *written* report about the image.

At London's Imperial College Hospital, some surgeons irate about being recorded covered up the hospital's cameras with surgical booties. Yet in a recent speech to his peers there, Dr. Krishna Moorthy got a standing ovation from his fellow surgeons (mostly younger ones) when he begged for more transparency—and more videotaped procedures. The upcoming generation of doctors is leading the way, saying this is what we would want if we were the patient. Telling the stories of his fifteen-year struggle to change the culture at his hospital, in a memorable tear-down-this-wall moment, Dr. Moorthy said impassionedly, "After fifteen years of cover-up, it's time for the shoe covers to come off."

CHAPTER 16

A New Generation for Honest Medicine

Throwing Instruments

As a resident, I saw a lot of surgeon tempers flare in the operating room. In an instant, a cordial surgeon could transform into an ogre, angry and unrelenting, creating a lasting culture of intimidation with a single outburst. Cursing at nurses, humiliating students, and scolding interns was commonplace. Occasionally I'd witness a surgeon throw an instrument on the floor, or even at another person, in a fit of rage. Rather than punish this behavior, the hospital rewarded it. Doctors who acted up tended to get what they wanted—the best nurse, the better room, the nicer locker. Ranting worked. The quieter doctors were often relegated to the leftover resources.

Thankfully, there is a new generation of doctors and nurses moving up through the ranks with little tolerance for the immature behavior once modeled by the surgical elite. The current generation of health professionals signed up for medicine on the understanding that there are rules: rules for behavior, mutual respect, and rules limiting their work week to a more humane schedule.

The new generation of students also wants to be more honest with patients than the last. They recognize the mistakes of twentieth-century medicine, are quick to point them out, and seek to start afresh. They also take a more holistic approach to healing; they are more attuned to the connection of mind and body, and willing to suggest nontraditional therapies. They're more forthright with patients about what they know and don't know. They believe in full disclosure and shared decision making and are more accepting of patients who refuse treatment. It's a gentler, more pragmatic generation of medical professionals; they are older, more diverse, more often married, and less male-dominated. Today, for the first time in history, women make up a majority of our medical-school class and surgical residency at Johns Hopkins, a milestone inconceivable to many in 1965, when Thomas Jefferson University medical school graduated its first woman doctor. Some have suggested that the female perspective helps to balance the male heritage of medicine's culture. Another difference in our profession is that for the first time, medical-school classes have more second-career students who entered medicine after being a teacher, businessperson, or nurse. They are more mature and are ready to object to things that just don't seem right, whether that is surgeons throwing temper tantrums or doctors withholding information from patients.

Having had no explanation of chiropractors when I was in medical school, I entered the hospital wards not knowing what exactly they do or whether it worked. I shrugged off this knowledge deficit until a patient asked me if she could see a chiropractor instead of having surgery for her neck. Scrambling back to the senior surgeon I worked with, I asked him what I should tell his patient. He told me he'd heard of a patient who died from a neck manipulation.

So I asked, "What exactly do you want me to tell her?" He replied, "Tell her she could have a rare complication from a chiropractic procedure and die."

I did. It worked—that is, it scared her off chiropractic treatment. Fortunately, she did not ask me to provide any comparative patient-outcome statistics. The party line for our group of trainees was to tell patients, "You could die," whenever they asked a question about options we weren't familiar with. I know now that in some cases, chiropractic treatment can be an effective alternative to surgery.

Today's medical students are not only able to speak to nontraditional therapies, they use them themselves. They take naturalist remedies, practice yoga or acupuncture, and have explored more nontraditional health modalities than most older doctors even know about. They refuse to glibly pass out the party line "You could die" and value honesty over allegiance to the medical hierarchy. Furthermore, they want to make a difference and believe in fixing the hazards of health care's delivery as much as they believe in curing disease.

When I interrupted medical school to attend graduate school for public health, I was seen as a black sheep. My medical-school dean at the time begged me not to do it and then told others I was getting a business degree even though I wasn't! Today, almost half of medical-school students and half of all interns and residents, including surgeons, express an interest in getting a master's degree in public health. From my vantage point, I am witnessing a generation eager to get at the root causes of our fragmented and uncoordinated system of care.

Most impressive, deans of medical schools are responding to the evolving attitudes of their students. Today if I threw a surgical instrument at a student, I'd probably get fired, which was not the case ten years ago when I witnessed such behavior. If I cursed at a student, I would likely get a lot of couch time in my boss's office. Bad behavior is no longer swept under the rug. Increasingly, hospitals are adopting anonymous online reporting systems so that nurses, students, and others can report disruptive behaviors or safety concerns. At some hospitals, like mine, such reports are investigated. When multiple reports confirm a bad actor, the dean or a powerful administrator can bring the disciplinary hammer down on that person.

The new, straight-shooting generation of students helps keep us all accountable. When I was a student, I was the equivalent of a private in the army, trained to follow orders with no questions asked. Not so with today's medical-school students. Every four weeks, I have a new pair of students shadowing me in every part of my job, providing a check on any potentially unethical or egregious behavior. While they may not have the expertise to know complex medical indications, they do know enough to know when something just doesn't look right, and they don't hesitate to query me.

A Surprising Conversation

Not too long ago, I had to work through the night trying to save a patient's life in an operation after an unexpected complication. It was physically draining surgery, and I was exhausted. The next morning my hair was up high, my beard was starting to sprout, and my clothes were awry. Then, while seeing patients in preparation for surgery, I wobbled, weak at the knees from standing for more than twenty-four hours. I couldn't help grinning as I remembered how an overworked visiting medical student doing an "audition rotation" once fell asleep while standing in a patient's room and slumped onto the very doctor he was trying to impress. I was also running on fumes and at risk for such a blunder. A Filipino nurse who usually compliments me as a sharp dresser smiled at my state of dishevelment. "Tough case last night, sir?"

Hearing the nurse's banter, my patient looked at me and asked point-blank, "Now, you got a good night's sleep last night—right, doctor?"

Her tone was jocular, but I could tell it was a serious question. I was silent, embarrassed, and confused as to how to respond. Quickly the patient picked up on my hesitation to answer and got anxious. This was a critical day for her, and I was not my best.

I decided on total honesty. I told her that I'd been up all night with an unexpected operation, and if she felt better rescheduling the surgery for a different date, then she should feel free. She opted to delay her surgery until the next day—probably wisely. Sometime after this episode, a research study came out showing an 83 percent increase in complications after elective surgery when

the surgeon was on call the night before and hadn't gotten ade-
quate sleep.[1] Whenever I share this with my nondoctor friends,
they respond in harmony: "You guys ought to know the consequences of bad sleep on your job!" In the past, like most doctors, I
would have smiled and said that working hard through sleep deprivation was part of a doctor's culture.

In a sign of the changing times, three Harvard doctors, Michael Nurok, Charles Czeisler, and Lisa Soleymani, defied the
entrenched cultural norms of the profession by writing in the *New
England Journal of Medicine* that surgeons ought to forthrightly
disclose to their elective-surgery patients when they've been up
all night. They argued that the patient should have the right to
choose whether to proceed with surgery or reschedule.[2] The piece
launched a national debate within medicine that split the surgical
community in half. Half argued vehemently that we need to treat
others as we would want to be treated. The other half argued that
patients don't need to know. Opponents of disclosure argued that
it would mark the beginning of a slippery slope that could lead
to surgeons having to disclose more about their mood and personal lives. Not surprisingly, those in favor of being honest with
patients were a strong and vocal group of mostly younger doctors.
I noticed that surgeons in training—and, notably, surgeons who
had been patients—led the battle cry in making the case for more
disclosure. At no time in my surgical education did I ever imagine that we as a community of doctors would be considering, even
debating, transparency at this level. This surprising national conversation is an indication that the culture of medicine is rapidly
changing.

The younger generation is also leading another charge. They
are talking more and more about "appropriateness" and custom-
izing care to individual patients. Even when textbook indications
are present, some procedures or medications can be inappropriate for frail, older patients. For example, a growing number of
doctors are questioning the propriety of screening a ninety-year-
old man for prostate cancer when such a cancer would likely take
ten to twenty years to take his life anyway. Blanket recommendations should be avoided, such as medication for everyone with a

slightly high blood pressure (systolic pressure of 150 to 160) or a high LDL cholesterol (over 100). If you made it to old age without medication for that blood pressure or with that cholesterol, you probably don't need to start now, even if generic national guidelines say to start treatment. Screening mammograms in certain age groups may cause more harm than good (triggering unnecessary surgery, not only for octogenarians but also for high schoolers). Medicine isn't always one size fits all, and as I noted earlier, there are cases when the best treatment is no treatment.[3] More doctors today understand this.

Medicine is an institution as old as humanity. Its traditions are as hierarchical as those of the royals. And for centuries, doctors have enhanced their authority with mystery, keeping the workings of their profession opaque. But I am convinced that the new generation of doctors is poised to usher in a revolution of transparency, open-mindedness, and honesty. This generational shift may be just what is needed for medicine to end the secrecy that has historically permeated our profession. With younger doctors taking the lead, the culture is ripe for transformation if we can capitalize on this moment and push for reform from within.

The signs of a new medical culture are multiplying. One example: For the first time in history, the American College of Surgeons and other doctors' groups are developing programs to address impaired physicians. This is a valuable step toward addressing the problem I discussed in chapter eight. Another example: Between writing chapters of this book, I attended the annual meeting of the Southern Surgical Association, a prestigious gathering of many of the country's top surgical leaders. There, I heard a remarkable keynote speech by incoming president Dr. J. Wayne Meredith, in which he condemned the way we "teach our new doctors to lie" in the first learning experience of their careers. He was criticizing the pervasive practice of surgeons indirectly pressuring interns to not record more than eighty hours on their weekly time card, even if they often work more than that. Dr. Meredith went on to address the issues of how doctors need to work together as a team and resist the incentives of the modern medical-industrial complex. Driven by the ultimate question—How would I want to be treated if I were a patient?—Dr. Meredith and other visionary figures are leading a culture change in health care.

CHAPTER 17

What Accountability Looks Like

BUSINESS LEADERS IN AMERICA ARE accountable for their earnings reports—by law. Thanks to the Sarbanes-Oxley Act, CEOs can now go to jail when they mislead the public about their performance. When President George H. W. Bush signed Sarbanes-Oxley into law, he described it as "the most far-reaching reforms of American business practices since the time of Franklin Delano Roosevelt."[1] Yet this accountability does not apply to the performance metrics of one fifth of the U.S. economy—health care.

Hospitals are not required to report their complication rates, readmission rates, or other standardized metrics of how they are performing. The only minor exception is a brand-new Medicare requirement for hospitals to begin reporting infection rates following a small subset of procedures. This provision is an early milestone for both the public and the doctors' groups that advocated for it. But it's hardly the overhaul we need. Even if modern medicine advances to the point at which we have full transparency on a broad scale, can the public trust self-reported data? Wall Street companies have independent auditors—oftentimes multiple auditors—go over their books to confirm the accuracy of their earnings reports. Yet only a small number of hospitals utilize independent reviewers to collect their patient-outcome statistics.

In the past few years, ways to make sure data collection is standardized and independent have matured thanks to the hard work of key professional physicians' groups, but hospitals have little

incentive to participate in these programs. Without the standardization that makes comparisons fair and accurate, true transparency
is unattainable. For example, hospitals that do a poor job self-
monitoring their infections get rewarded for having low rates, and
conversely hospitals with close patient follow-up and independent
nurses to monitor infections are punished for capturing more infections via higher reported rates. A marketplace of self-reporting with
no accountability can mislead patients rather than empower them.

People use corporate-earnings information to make personal investment decisions. So too should the public have reliable hospital-
performance information to make informed decisions about their
medical care.

In our current medical marketplace, where key performance
statistics are largely kept secret, a hospital CEO can know that his
or her hospital has an exceptionally high complication rate for a
particular service, but have little incentive to address the problem
since the customer is in the dark. In fact, the hospital is financially
rewarded for continuing to provide a dangerous service. In other
words, a hospital can knowingly sell a service it knows to be far
more dangerous than the national average, and continue to sell
that service without having to answer to anyone. Believe it or not,
that's our system. When we learned that Goldman Sachs had been
selling financial products to the public that they were internally
calling "crap" and were also betting against, the public was outraged, and members of Congress cried foul in a heated hearing on
Capitol Hill. With hospitals, the stakes are even higher—patient
lives—yet our standards of disclosure are lower than those for
Wall Street.

Dangers

It seems that policy makers are testing the waters, waiting to see
if the public wants more transparency in health care. Most of the
current discussions focus on public reporting of infection rates
for a few select types of surgery. While the current proposals are
a start, infection rates are only one tiny sliver of the pie. Don't be

misled. A few limited metrics won't tell you about the quality of care or the hospital's performance as a whole. Requiring only some infection rates to be public can actually be counterproductive. Hospitals take their public image so seriously that they have been known to redirect all their efforts to the single metric that's being made public, neglecting other important issues. Focusing on only one can be very dangerous.

For example, one of the more well-known measures cardiologists have developed is door-to-balloon time—the interval between when a patient says he or she has chest pain to when an angioplasty balloon is inflated inside that patient's heart vessel, letting more blood pass through the blockage. Door-to-balloon time represents how efficient a hospital is in taking the patient from the ER door to the surgical suite for this potentially lifesaving procedure. It was devised as a measure of quality of care that would be standardized, feasible, and fair. (Tampering with the recorded time of the nurse's intake note or the angioplasty report would represent a serious case of fraud, and such blatant misreporting would be highly unlikely.) So the door-to-balloon-time metric sounded like an excellent way to measure quality of a hospital.

At least that's what I thought, until I heard one hospital was being less precise about which patients underwent balloon procedures, allegedly to rush them through the process to look good on the metric. Furthermore, a study later found that faster door-to-balloon times may not translate into better patient outcomes.[2] The catch is that while angioplasty can be a lifesaving procedure, it can also be an unnecessary and expensive one. Without a sister metric to show the *appropriateness* of angioplasty, hospitals were so heavily incentivized to rush patients through the emergency room to the angioplasty suite, they began to pay less attention to whether the patient really needed it done! Some hospitals with the shortest times achieved them because they weren't bothering to decide who really needed an angioplasty. They were overballooning as a result of trying too hard to look good to the public on their door-to-balloon-time metric. The problem was that the metric was not comprehensive. It looked at only one aspect of care while ignoring many other important ones.

In 2005, British Airways learned the lesson of one-dimensional metrics the hard way. Passengers on a British Airways Boeing 747 from Los Angeles to London heard a loud explosion, looked out the window, and observed one of the engines in flames. A copilot came out of the cockpit and walked the length of the rattling hull to take a look. An air-traffic controller at LAX radioed in, "Speed-bird 268 heavy, it appears you have flames coming out of either your number-one or number-two engine," and sat back expecting that the pilot would request to land. Instead the pilot said he'd be calling British Airways to discuss what to do.[3]

Remarkably, with 351 passengers and eighteen crew members on board, British Airways decided the plane should continue on to its destination, London. The pilot radioed the LAX air-traffic controller back, "We just decided we want to set off on our flight-plan route and get as far as we can . . . thanks for your help, cheers." The plane crossed the United States at a lower altitude and a speed 12 percent slower than normal due to increased drag from the dead engine. On approach to the East Coast, the crew had to decide whether to risk crossing the Atlantic for London despite the faster rate of fuel consumption. They decided to go for it. Finally, just shy of London, the captain declared an emergency requiring a landing in Manchester, England, due to concerns there was not enough fuel. Luckily, all passengers and crew landed safely.

Before the incident, the European Union introduced financial incentives for on-time arrivals under which all arrivals over five hours late would result in airlines compensating passengers a total of $275,000. Pilot groups fought the rule on grounds of safety, but lost. Pilots feared that these incentives would encourage pilots to cut safety corners. Which is just what happened.

On-time arrivals are only one way to measure good performance. A more comprehensive set of metrics would include input from air-traffic controllers, mechanical teams, and the very telling employee-safety-culture surveys, among others. It turns out that this was not the first time this happened at British Airways. Other similar incidents had occurred in preceding years. Following this last and most highly scrutinized event, British Airways got the point and addressed the practice. For both cardiologists and British Airways pilots, focusing on just one metric proved to be at the expense of other processes important to a quality outcome.

The Movement from Within

Up to this point, transparency has been driven by forward-thinking doctors who know what it could do for our health care system and think New York State's successful experiment with heart-surgery outcomes could be conducted on a larger scale.

Doctors' societies have now developed irrefutable metrics of performance for their own specialties that account for complications and complexities, incorporating data about how doctors and hospitals have gamed the system. Independent reviews check the data to prevent distortion and misreporting. Any good doctor wants his or her patients to choose their care with meaningful information. Doctors also want to practice in a collaborative environment unencumbered by meaningless bureaucracy and soul-corroding ethical dilemmas.

Doctors need to press their own administrations on transparency. Patient-advocacy groups can't work against the system alone. Doctors understand the science and have developed nonbiased methodologies for tracking quality, and a younger generation is already expressing a distaste for the old way of doing things.

Nurses, too, play a central role as mediators between patients and the rest of the hospital system. As such they are especially important to the transparency movement. Many nurses' associations are already making transparency one of their top priorities. The Association of periOperative Registered Nurses, with its forty-thousand-plus membership, has campaigned to encourage nurses to speak up when something doesn't look right. The American Nurses Association has also focused on more teamwork in patient safety.

The American College of Surgeons recently announced that improving quality of surgical care in the United States will be its top priority. Part of the initiative is a series of programs to screen and help impaired physicians and to create new standards of accreditation and bedside care. The organization also endorses full public reporting of patient outcomes. Several other organizations are doing the same. For the first time in American medicine, there is grassroots interest from within to make doctors and the hospitals they work in more accountable.

What Change Might Look Like: The Online Dashboard

Just as a car has a dashboard of relevant, easy-to-read data, so too should hospitals provide the same. The effect would likely be a global reduction in patient harm and a rise in customer satisfaction. Patient-outcome reports need to include comprehensive outcomes of how well patients do, not just infection rates for a few select procedures. Specifically, for every hospital in a particular area, a consumer should be able to look up the following hospital outcomes by medical condition. These metrics need to be user-friendly and centralized for consumers to access easily. What follows are concrete measures for tracking hospital performance.

1. Bouncebacks
A consumer should be able to look up the percentage of hospitalized patients who are readmitted to a hospital within ninety days, categorized by the discharging diagnosis. Doctors call this the bounceback rate. For my area of medicine, pancreas surgery, it's about 20 to 40 percent. Readmission rates are already actively collected at most U.S. hospitals. New formulas designed to mathematically adjust for patient disease complexity can yield a score relative to the national average.

In addition to reporting readmission rates, hospitals should also report their average length of stay for each medical condition category. Having only one of these two metrics could be misleading. While some baseline rate of readmission is expected, a hospital with an unusually high readmission rate might be sending its patients out the door too early, providing lower-quality care, and giving patients poor instructions at the time of discharge.

2. Complication Rates

A complication is any unexpected adverse event that develops during or after a medical treatment or procedure. Consumers should be able to go online and enter their medical condition or proposed operation and review the hospitalwide complication rate for that treatment or procedure. Specifically, consumers should be able to see how frequently the seven major complication types occur: respiratory, cardiovascular, bleeding, wound/infectious, gastrointestinal/malnutrition, kidney, and neurologic. In addition, consumers should have access to risk-adjusted mortality statistics, as I do at my hospital.

The science of measuring complications has matured: Doctors' associations have developed and now endorse fair ways to collect this information using standardized doctor-authored definitions for complications. In some of these outcome-measurement collaboratives, independent nurses use protocols to comb through charts, scan electronic records and billing information, and call patients to find out if they have had a complication. This data can easily be entered through a web-based portal and sorted by algorithms that adjust complication rates for condition complexity and disease. This should occur at all hospitals, and the results should be accessible on your computer or smart phone.

3. Never Events

Never events are things that should absolutely never happen in a hospital. Different from complications, which cannot be completely eliminated, never events are by definition avoidable. They include leaving sponges or instruments inside a patient after surgery, performing the wrong operation or the right one on the wrong side or the wrong patient, or death during elective surgery in a healthy patient. These catastrophes should simply never occur. Never events sound shocking, but most every hospital in the country, including every hospital I have ever worked in, has had *at least* a couple every year. Public reporting would enable patients to see which hospitals rarely have a never event and which have them often. The public is rightly concerned by this persistent problem in medicine. Public scrutiny of hospital never-event rates would prioritize prevention efforts, since each never event would no longer simply mean a quiet monetary settlement with a patient—it could mean a costly PR nightmare.

4. Safety-Culture Scores

Approximately fifteen hundred hospitals administer the safety survey to their doctors, nurses, and other health care workers. The percent of hospital workers that say "yes" to the following three questions should be made public:

- "Would you have your operation at the hospital in which you work?"
- "Do you feel comfortable speaking up when you have a safety concern?"
- "Does the teamwork here promote doing what's right for the patient?"

This information may be more comprehensive and revealing than any other metric in health care. Ways for the surveys to be administered are standardized to ensure a fair playing field for comparisons between hospitals. If you had access to this information, you would likely avoid the hospital at which only a quarter of its staff would go for their own care, and choose hospitals that have a strong culture of safety and teamwork. This would incentivize hospitals to invest in an aspect of medical care undervalued for too long.

5. Hospital Volumes

Hospitals should be reporting how many patients with a particular type of medical condition they treat and how many of each type of surgery they perform annually (or totals over a multiyear period clearly marked for the number of years). There is no reason for hospitals not to provide the number of pneumonia, stroke, and shoulder problems they treat each year, which presents no delicate issues concerning individual doctor reputations. A breast-cancer patient, for instance, ought to be able to find centers that do a lot of operations of that type (including superior DIEP reconstructions versus standard reconstruction procedures). The number of babies delivered, including C-section rate, should be made public so expecting mothers can be properly informed. Similarly, every hospital should report what percent of their operations are performed using minimally invasive surgery versus traditional open surgery. Consumers can then make their own comparisons.

6. Transparent Records, Open Notes, and Video Recording

Consumers should be able to find out which hospitals participate in programs that streamline access to written and video records. Hospitals that have family- and patient-centered programs or policies mandating full disclosures of all drug- and device-related financial conflicts of interest should be easy to find for prospective patients researching hospitals. Currently, you need to make dozens of phone calls to find out if these programs are in place.

New Advocates for Change

Ask any businessperson why health care is hemorrhaging cash and you'll be told that there's no measurable product. Money is poured into the system with no record of how it's performing. This is very unusual in America. Every industry in our society and every service on which money is spent is judged by what you get in return—except health care. The medical system collects billions of dollars from the government, private companies, insurers, and individuals, yet it provides few practical metrics of performance. The business dictum "If you can't measure it, you can't improve it" applies directly to the current health care mess.

There is reason to believe this is starting to change. The Leapfrog Group for Patient Safety is a group of business leaders fed up with health care's lack of transparency. It has developed its own standards, based on the latest medical evidence, that it asks hospitals to meet. These include performing a minimum number of each type of complex operation in order to receive its seal as safe, and it is becoming a seal of approval that hospitals desire. What started as whispered frustration among top business leaders has become a nationwide movement to reform health care. The Leapfrog Group exemplifies how a small but influential group can demand, and get, common-sense change in health care.

Other groups, such as the Institute for Healthcare Improvement (IHI), a national resource center created to help hospitals perform better, focus on reducing error rates and implementing best practices by redesigning care to make it safer. They have likely saved hundreds of thousands of lives by walking hospitals through error-prevention strategies and teaching models that work in the national learning forum they host.

Pascal Metrics is another quick responder to the health care crisis. They administer the safety-culture survey at hospitals and report the results back cogently so that hospitals can see where they stand nationally. Pascal and other organizations are also creating hospital computer systems to detect preventable patient harms before they occur. These smart computers use various warning flags, or "triggers," that in certain mathematical combinations indicate that something bad is about to happen to a patient. These triggers include an abnormally long operation, a routine surgery unexpectedly requiring an overnight stay, a new lab result of a low oxygen level, or a request for a cardiologist outside of the cardiology unit.[4] Using a sophisticated model that monitors an array of data from afar, these computer systems sense an escalating risk for medical disasters in real time and alert a special prevention team to respond immediately before the disaster happens. Preventing dangerous and expensive complications before they occur is one of the benefits of the many promising innovations being designed to make medicine safer.

Some hospitals are also stepping up. A small group of them—Washington University hospital in St. Louis, the Cleveland Clinic, Johns Hopkins, and even the same hospital in which I first witnessed Hodad—have expressed a willingness to publicly report some of the main outcomes that they routinely collect. Some states have also begun to experiment constructively with transparency in medicine. Minnesota has begun reporting hospital complications online for certain conditions. At some point, demand from the public may become impossible for administrators to ignore, as consumers and insurers start to wonder what it is that the non-disclosing hospitals are trying to hide.

Nonetheless, so far much of the most effective pressure for change has come from patients—or, sadly, from their bereaved family members. David and Patty Skolnik were singlehandedly able to convince the Colorado legislature to reform its state medical board. After their twenty-two-year-old son, Michael, underwent unnecessary brain surgery, he developed serious complications and became partially blind and disabled for three miserable years, then developed a seizure and died from yet another medical mistake made at that time. Too late, the Skolniks found that their son's neurosurgeon had a dark past with many problems in other states. Patty vowed that no other family would suffer what she had endured. She championed a reform law to increase transparency among Colorado doctors—named the Michael Skolnik Medical Transparency Act in her late son's honor. Patty also got Colorado to expand the data available on the website of the state medical board so that now it is the most comprehensive in the country.

The Skolniks' tragic story shows how the consumers of health care can make a difference. I believe that our modern-day corporate hospitals will respond if patients demand accountability. Even small victories can build into larger ones. After her legislative success, Patty began a small group called Colorado Citizens for Accountability that gained so much momentum it is now a global organization called Citizens for Patient Safety (citizensforpatient safety.org), providing resources for patients, advancing transparency legislation in other states, and training doctors and students.

Conclusion

IN THE PAST CENTURY, MEDICINE learned to use an incredibly powerful tool that has saved lives and improved the efficacy of treatments and the quality of care. That tool was data. The revolution it made possible was called evidence-based medicine. No doctor, nurse, or health care executive today would ignore the value of carefully collected data in determining the best ways to treat patients.

Yet even as our system relies on evidence to function, we fail to make the same tool available to patients who are confronting decisions of critical, even life-and-death importance. The evidence-based revolution has already transformed medicine for the better. Now we need a transparency revolution.

Transparency has the power not just to improve the experience of patients, but to transform the business of health care in America. Congress should make transparency a condition of Medicare reimbursement and other types of funding. Lawmakers, Medicare officials, and some state medical boards have been expressing interest. Now that we do have reliable ways to measure performance, the time has come for action.

When I speak around the country on how medicine has become so fragmented, uncoordinated, and costly, people often ask me what they can do about it. My answer to them is to insist on transparency. And support the movement. Medicine is a cloister, but it's still a business that depends on the public. Patients are the consumer, and no business wants its clients to take their business elsewhere. Some hospitals and even individual doctors are taking a simple transparency pledge to participate in public reporting of outcomes, disclose all conflicts of interest, streamline patient access to records, and disclose mistakes as soon as they learn about them. I have taken this pledge, and I've posted it on the website for this book, unaccountablebook.com.

If you want to become a part of this effort, write your local hospital CEO and board members, encouraging them to make their outcomes public information and to take a transparency pledge. Then encourage them to market their hospital with their strong performance on comprehensive metrics and a promise to be transparent at the bedside. Legislators and governors are also starting to listen to their constituents on this issue—especially to hear the other side to recent lobbying efforts to block public reporting. And although the general public may not appreciate the movement from within, more and more doctors are rising up to demand that modern medicine be responsive to the public.

Transparency in America would also be a healthy complement to proposals for much-needed tort reform, which aims to reduce the high costs of malpractice liability from frivolous lawsuits. In a truly transparent system in which patients could easily find quality care, we would see fewer complications and fewer lawsuits.

The increasing cost of health care is an unsustainable burden on American families, businesses, and government budgets, to the point that it is now the leading driver of the growing national debt. Yet I rarely hear "experts" speak to its root cause—the accountability problem. When I listen to health care gurus propose overhauling the health care system with new ways to finance it, I often feel that they are tragically off the mark. The simplest, most economical solution to the problems of our complex system is to *empower patients with information.*

Political partisans can debate the role of government in fixing health care, but for either public or private approaches to work, transparency is the crucial prerequisite. And openness and accountability are values that Americans across the political spectrum agree on. The reforms advocated in this book are neither conservative nor liberal. To make transparency effective, government, insurance companies, hospitals, and doctors' groups must play a role in making fair and accurate reports available to the public. Add by doing so, it will unleash the power of the free market to create positive change. When hospitals have to compete on a level playing field, all of them will be forced to improve how they serve their patients.

There will be another important benefit to transparency: It can restore the respect of the public in what many perceive has become a secretive, even arrogant industry. With accountability, medicine can address the cost crisis, deliver safer care, and earn once more the trust of the communities we serve.

Acknowledgments

In my eleven years of education and training after college, there have been many doctors and health policy experts who have mentored me. Characteristic to all, they do not like credit, but I would like to acknowledge them. Foremost are Dr. Andy Warshaw and Dr. Carlos Fernandez-del Castillo, two highly skilled surgeons whose humble attitudes and deep compassion inspired me to become a surgeon despite the problems of modern medicine. I am also grateful to Dr. Stephen R. T. Evans, Dr. David Bates, and Dr. Geno Merli, who taught me to always tell the truth and that doctoring is a privilege. Drs. David Hemenway and Harvey Fineberg have also encouraged me to be aware of medicine's unique subculture as I reside in it. They encouraged me as a medical student to think differently and to consider researching medical errors in the same way we would research a disease to find its causes and its cure.

I am deeply grateful to Peter Ginna for his advice and guidance, and to Lynn Chu, Glen Hartley, Laura Phillips, and Jen Dwyer, who helped me shape this book. Pete Beatty, Michelle Blankenship, and Laura Keefe similarly helped the effort tremendously. I also would like to thank Stephanie Fey Desmon, Gary Stephens, and JoAnn Rodgers, who have worked hard to translate our research on quality and safety into a message that can improve health care.

I have been greatly inspired by Heather Lyu, Michol Cooper, Andrew Ibrahim, Linda Jin, and the many medical students, nurses, and policy advocates who after learning about this movement dedicated a great deal of time to promote a national conversation about accountability in medicine. They have joined a grassroots effort that continues to grow from the deep convictions of health care workers and patients and their family members. I also would like to thank Drs. Bruce Hall, Clifford Ko, Michael Henderson, Karen Richards, and David Shahian, who have helped elevate the field of quality medical care into a formal science. Finally I would like to thank the Halsted residents of the Johns Hopkins Hospital for their enthusiasm in advancing the great heritage of the Hippocratic oath in their practice of medicine and the art of teaching it to others.

Notes

Introduction

1. C. P. Landrigan, "Temporal Trends in Rates of Patient Harm Resulting from Medical Care," *New England Journal of Medicine* 363, no. 22 (2010): 2124–34.

Chapter 1: Dr. Hodad and the Raptor

1. Kevin Sack and Marjorie Connelly, "In Poll, Wide Support for Government-Run Health," *New York Times*, June 20, 2009.

Chapter 2: Danger Zones

1. M. A. Makary, J. B. Sexton et al., "Patient Safety in Surgery," *Annals of Surgery* 243, no. 5 (2006): 628–35. See also M. A. Makary, J. B. Sexton et al. "Teamwork in the Operating Room: Frontline Perspectives among Hospitals and Operating Room Personnel," *Anesthesiology* 105, no. 5 (2006): 877–84. All safety-culture charts are from these studies.

2. Committee on Quality of Health Care in America and the Institute of Medicine with eds. L. T. Kohn, J. M. Corrigan, M. S. Donaldson, *To Err Is Human: Building a Safer Health System* (Washington, D.C.: National Academy Press, 2000).

3. D. T. Huang et al., "Intensive Care Unit Safety Culture and Outcomes: A U.S. Multicenter Study," *International Journal for Quality in Health Care* 22, no. 3 (2010):151–61; A. B. Haynes, Safe Surgery Saves Lives Study Group et al., "Changes in Safety Attitude and Relationship to Decreased Postoperative Morbidity and Mortality Following Implementation of a Checklist-based Surgical Safety Intervention," *BMJ Quality and Safety* 20, no. 1 (2011): 102–07.

4. Author interview with Dr. Guy Clifton, August 22, 2011.
5. J. B. Dimick et al., "Who Pays for Poor Surgical Quality? Building a Business Case for Quality Improvement," *Journal of the American College of Surgeons* 202, no. 6 (2006): 933–37.

Chapter 3: The New York Experiment

1. M. R. Chassin, "Achieving and Sustaining Improved Quality: Lessons from New York State and Cardiac Surgery," *Health Affairs* 21, no. 4 (2002): 40–51.
2. Ibid.
3. Society of Thoracic Surgeons, "STS Public Reporting Online," last modified 2012, sts.org/quality-research-patient-safety/sts-public -reporting-online.
4. P. S. Romano et al., "Impact of Public Reporting of Coronary Artery Bypass Graft Surgery Performance Data on Market Share, Mortality, and Patient Selection," *Medical Care* 49, no. 12 (2011): 1118–25.
5. Author interview with Dr. William R. Brody.
6. Mark Benjamin, "Military Injustice," *Salon*, June 7, 2005.

Chapter 4: The Supersurgeon and the Shah

1. L. Morgenstern, "The Shah's Spleen: Its Impact on History," *Journal of the American College of Surgeons* 212, no. 12 (2011): 260–68.
2. David Harris, *The Crisis: The President, the Prophet, and the Shah—1979 and the Coming of Militant Islam* (New York: Little, Brown and Company, 2004).
3. E. L. Hannan et al. "The Decline in Coronary Artery Bypass Graft Surgery Mortality in New York State: The Role of Surgeon Volume," *Journal of the American Medical Association* 273, no. 3 (1995): 209–13.

Chapter 5: "How I Like to Do It"

1. Atul Gawande, "The Cost Conundrum," *New Yorker*, June 1, 2009.
2. John Carreyrou and Maurice Tamman, "A Device to Kill Cancer, Lift Revenue," *Wall Street Journal*, December 7, 2010.

Chapter 6: Navigating the System

1. Kaiser Family Foundation, "New National Survey: Are Patients Ready to Be Health Care Consumers?" October 28, 1996, http://www.kff.org/insurance/1203-qualrel.cfm.

Chapter 7: Tap the Power of Patient Outcomes

1. E. A. Codman, *A Study in Hospital Efficiency* (reprinted by the Joint Commission on Accreditation of Healthcare Organizations Press, 1996).

2. S. F. Khuri, et al., "The Department of Veterans Affairs' NSQIP: The First National, Validated, Outcome-based, Risk-adjusted, and Peer-controlled Program for the Measurement and Enhancement of the Quality of Surgical Care," *Annals of Surgery* 228, no. 4 (1998): 491–507.

3. O. D. Guillamondegui et al., "Using the National Surgical Quality Improvement Program and the Tennessee Surgical Quality Collaborative to Improve Surgical Outcomes," *Journal of the American College of Surgeons* 214, no. 4 (2012): 709–14.

4. Author interview with Robert Herbold, June 9, 2011.

Chapter 8: Impaired Physicians

1. L. N. Dyrbye et al., "Work/Home Conflict and Burnout among Academic Internal Medicine Physicians," *Archives of Internal Medicine* 171, no. 13 (2011): 1207–09; J. E. Wallace et al., "Physician Wellness: A Missing Quality Indicator," *The Lancet* 374, no. 9702 (2009): 1714–21.

2. T. D. Shanafelt et al., "Burnout and Career Satisfaction among American Surgeons," *Annals of Surgery* 250, no. 3 (2009): 463–71.

3. John Fauber, "Cardiologist Who Revealed Echo Errors Out of a Job," January 14, 2011, http://www.medpagetoday.com/Cardiology/Atherosclerosis/24337.

4. William Heisel, "Maine Welcomes Psychiatrist with Fraud Conviction and Drug Abuse Concerns," Reporting on Health blog, September 1, 2010, http://www.reportingonhealth.org/node/9476.

5. A. Levine et al., "State Medical Boards Fail to Discipline Doctors with Hospital Actions Against Them," *Public Citizen Report*, March 15, 2011, www.citizen.org/documents/1937.pdf.

6. Cheryl W. Thompson, "After Stealing Drugs, Doctor Goes to Rehab: Anesthesiologist Licensed to Practice in Several States" *Washington Post*, April 10, 2005.

7. Toby Bilanow, "When Older Doctors Put Patients at Risk," *New York Times*, Well blog, January 24, 2011, http://well.blogs.nytimes.com/2011/01/24/when-older-doctors-put-patients-at-risk.

Chapter 9: Medical Mistakes

1. C. P. Landrigan et al., "Temporal Trends in Rates of Patient Harm Resulting from Medical Care," *New England Journal of Medicine* 363, no. 22 (2010): 2124–34.

2. Dina ElBoghdady, "Some Doctors Try to Squelch Online Reviews," *Washington Post*, January 28, 2012.

3. Author interview with Alan Levine.

4. D. Josefson et al., "Transplants from Live Patients Scrutinized after Donor's Death," *British Medical Journal* 324, no. 7340 (2002): 754.

5. Scott Allen, "With Work, Dana-Farber Learns from '94 Mistakes," *Boston Globe*, November 30, 2004.

6. I. Philibert et al. for the members of the ACGME Work Group on Resident Duty Hours, "New Requirements for Resident Duty Hours," *Journal of the American Medical Association* 288, no. 9 (2002): 1112–14.

7. Alison Leigh Cowan, "Mount Sinai May Resume a Liver Transplant Program," *New York Times*, March 22, 2003.

8. Lydia Polgreen, "Transplant Chief at Mt. Sinai Quits Post in Wake of Inquiry," *New York Times*, September 7, 2002.

9. Darshak Sanghavi, "The Phantom Menace of Sleep-Deprived Doctors," *New York Times Magazine*, August 5, 2011.

10. Denise Grady, "Four Transplant Recipients Contract H.I.V.," *New York Times*, November 13, 2007.

Chapter 10: Ask Before You Give

1. Gilbert M. Gaul, "Children's Hospitals Pay Millions to CEOs," *Fort Worth Star-Telegram*, September 26, 2011.

2. Ibid.

3. Forbes.com, "The 200 Largest U.S. Charities," November 17, 2010, http://www.forbes.com/lists/2010/14/charity-10_Childrens-Hospital-Boston_CH0036.html.

4. Forbes.com, "The 200 Largest U.S. Charities," November 17, 2010, http://www.forbes.com/2009/11/23/charitable-giving-gates-foundation-personal-finance-charity-09-intro.html.

Chapter 11: Eat What You Kill

1. John Carreyrou and Tom McGinty, "Medicare Records Reveal Troubling Trail of Surgeries," *Wall Street Journal*, March 29, 2011.

2. John Carreyrou and Tom McGinty, "Top Spine Surgeons Reap Royalties, Medicare Bounty," *Wall Street Journal*, December 20, 2010.

3. Ibid.

4. Shannon Brownlee, *Overtreated: Why Too Much Medicine Is Making Us Sicker and Poorer* (New York: Bloomsbury, 2007).

5. J. P. Neoptolemos et al., "A Randomized Trial of Chemoradiotherapy and Chemotherapy after Resection of Pancreatic Cancer," *New England Journal of Medicine* 350, no. 12 (2004): 1200–10.

6. Matthew Heineman and Susan Froemke, *Escape Fire: The Fight to Rescue American Healthcare*, (2012, no distributor).

7. E. J. Emanuel et al., "Chemotherapy Use among Medicare Beneficiaries at the End of Life," *Annals of Internal Medicine* 138, no. 8 (2003): 639–43.

8. Andrew Pollack, "Genentech Offers Secret Rebates for Eye Drug," *New York Times*, November 3, 2010.

9. Robert Little, "Patients Learn They Might Have Unneeded Stents," *Baltimore Sun*, January 15, 2010.

10. Ron Winslow and John Carreyrou, "Heart Treatment Overused," *Wall Street Journal*, July 6, 2011.

11. Paul S. Chan et al., "Appropriateness of Percutaneous Coronary Intervention," *Journal of the American Medical Association* 306, no. 1 (2011): 53–61.

12. Jon Kamp, "Heart-Device Guidelines Not Often Met, Study Says," *Wall Street Journal*, January 5, 2011.

Chapter 12: The All-American Robot

1. Intuitive Surgical Inc., *2010 Annual Report* (Sunnyvale, CA: Intuitive Surgical, Inc., 2001).

2. A. M. Ibrahim et al., unpublished research, Johns Hopkins University, 2011.

3. A. M. Ibrahim and M. A. Makary, "Robot-Assisted Surgery and Health Care Costs," *New England Journal of Medicine* 363, no. 22 (2010): 2175–76.

4. G. I. Barbash and S. A. Glied, "New Technology and Health Care Costs: The Case of Robotic-Assisted Surgery," *New England Journal of Medicine* 363, no. 8 (2010): 701–04.

5. Ibid.

6. L. Jin et al., "Robotic Surgery Claims on U.S. Hospital Websites," *Journal on Healthcare Quality* 33, no. 6 (2011): 48–52.

7. John Carreyrou, "Surgical Robot Examined in Injuries," *Wall Street Journal*, May 4, 2010.

8. Patient-Centered Outcomes Research Institute, "What We Do," last modified September 14, 2011, http://www.pcori.org/what-we-do/pcor.

Chapter 13: Drivers of Culture

1. Mayo Clinic, "Mayo Clinic Mission and Values," last modified November 10, 2011, http://www.mayoclinic.org/about/missionvalues.html.

2. Memo from R. M. Boisjoly to R. K. Lund, July 31, 1985, Presidential Commission on the Space Shuttle *Challenger* Accident, Archives II Reference Section (Civilian), Textual Archives Services Division (NWCT2R[C]), National Archives at College Park, MD (online version at http://arcweb.archives.gov).

3. M. A. Makary et al., "Operating Room Briefings: Working on the Same Page," *Joint Commission Journal on Quality and Patient Safety* 32, no. 6 (2006): 351–55. M. A. Makary et al., "Operating Room Briefings and Wrong-Site Surgery," *Journal of the American College of Surgeons* 204, no. 2 (2007): 236–43.

4. Lawrence K. Altman, "Doctors Discuss Transplant Mistake," *New York Times*, February 22, 2003.

5. M. A. Makary et al.,"Needlestick Injuries among Surgeons in Training," *New England Journal of Medicine* 356, no. 26 (2007): 2693–99.

6. M. A. Makary et al., "Operating Room Teamwork among Physicians and Nurses: Teamwork in the Eye of the Beholder," *Journal of the American College of Surgeons* 202, no. 5 (2006): 746–52.

7. A. S. Klein and P. M. Forni, "Barbers of Civility," *Archives of Surgery* 146, no. 7 (2011): 774–77.

8. J. B. Sexton et al., "Teamwork in the Operating Room: Frontline Perspectives among Hospitals and Operating Room Personnel," *Anesthesiology* 105, no. 5 (2006): 877–84.

9. M. A. Makary et al., "Operating Room Briefings: Working on the Same Page"; M. A. Makary et al., "Operating Room Briefings and Wrong-Site Surgery"; and S. Nundy et al., "Impact of Preoperative Briefings on Operating Room Delays," *Archives of Surgery* 143, no. 11 (2008): 1068–72.

10. A. B. Haynes, et al. for the Safe Surgery Saves Lives Study Group, "A Surgical Safety Checklist to Reduce Morbidity and Mortality in a Global Population," *New England Journal of Medicine* 360, no. 5 (2009): 491–99.

11. E. Wick et al., "Implementation of a Comprehensive Unit-based Safety Program (CUSP) to Reduce Surgical Site Infections," *Journal of the American College of Surgeons* (forthcoming).

12. D. T. Huang et al., "Intensive Care Unit Safety Culture and Outcomes: A U.S. Multicenter Study," *International Journal for Quality in Health Care* 22, no. 3 (2010): 151–61. M. Cooper and M. A. Makary, "A Comprehensive Unit-Based Safety Program (CUSP) in Surgery: Im-

proving Quality through Transparency," *Surgical Clinics of North America* 92, no. 1 (2012): 51–63.

Chapter 14: Healthonomics

1. J. Tse et al., "How Accurate Is the Electronic Health Record? A Pilot Study Evaluating Information Accuracy in a Primary Care Setting," *Studies in Health Technology and Informatics* 168 (2011): 158–64.
2. M. Staroselsky et al., "Improving Electronic Health Record (EHR) Accuracy and Increasing Compliance with Health Maintenance Clinical Guidelines through Patient Access and Input," *International Journal of Medical Informatics* 75, nos. 10–11 (2006): 693–700.
3. D. Syin et al., "Publication Bias in Surgery," *Journal of Surgical Research* 143, no. 1 (2007): 88–93.
4. C. Charles et al., "Shared Decision-Making in the Medical Encounter: What Does It Mean? (or It Takes at Least Two to Tango)," *Social Science & Medicine* 44, no. 5 (1997): 681–92.

Chapter 15: Candid Cameras

1. Larry Copeland, "Research: Red-light Cameras Work," *USA Today*, February 15, 2007.
2. Author interview with Dr. Douglas Rex.
3. D. K. Rex et al., "The Impact of Videorecording on the Quality of Colonoscopy Performance: A Pilot Study," *American Journal of Gastroenterology* 105, no. 11 (2010): 2312–17.
4. M. Raghavendra and D. K. Rex, "Patient Interest in Video Recording of Colonoscopy: A Survey," *World Journal of Gastroenterology* 16, no. 4 (2010): 458–61.
5. A. S. Klein and P. M. Forni, "Barbers of Civility," *Archives of Surgery* 146, no. 7 (2011): 774–77.
6. Tina Rosenberg, "An Electronic Eye on Hospital Hand-Washing," *New York Times*, Opinionator blog, November 24, 2011, http://opinionator.blogs.nytimes.com/2011/11/24/an-electronic-eye-on-hospital-hand-washing.
7. Joseph Brownstein, "Rhode Island Hospital Fined for Fifth Surgery Error in Two Years," ABCNews.com, November 4, 2009, http://abcnews.go.com/Health/rhode-island-hospital-fined-surgery-error-years/story?id=8988619.
8. P. Lee, S. Regenbogen, and A. A. Gawande, "How Many Surgical Procedures Will Americans Experience in an Average Lifetime? Evidence from Three States," http://www.mcacs.org/abstracts/2008/P15.cgi.

9. World Health Organization, "New Scientific Evidence Supports WHO Findings: A Surgical Safety Checklist Could Save Hundreds of Thousands of Lives," http://www.who.int/patientsafety/safesurgery/checklist_saves_lives/en/index.html.

Chapter 16: A New Generation for Honest Medicine

1. M. Nurok et al., "Sleep Deprivation, Elective Surgical Procedures, and Informed Consent," *New England Journal of Medicine* 363, no. 27 (2010): 2577–79.
2. Ibid.
3. Sharon Begley, "One Word that Can Save Your Life: No!" *Newsweek*, August 14, 2011.

Chapter 17: What Accountability Looks Like

1. U.S. Congress. *Sarbanes-Oxley Act of 2002*. Public Law 107–204. 107th Congress. *Congressional Record* 148 (July 30, 2002).
2. A. Flynn et al., "Trends in Door-to-Balloon Time and Mortality in Patients with ST-Elevation Myocardial Infarction Undergoing Primary Percutaneous Coronary Intervention," *Archives of Internal Medicine* 170, no. 20 (2010): 1842–9.
3. Scott McCartney, "After Engine Blew, Deciding to Fly On 'As Far as We Can,' " *Wall Street Journal*, September 23, 2006.
4. F. A. Griffin et al., "Detection of Adverse Events in Surgical Patients Using the Trigger Tool Approach," *Quality and Safety in Health Care* 17, no. 4 (2008): 253–58; D. C. Classen et al. " 'Global Trigger Tool' Shows that Adverse Events in Hospitals May Be Ten Times Greater than Previously Measured," *Health Affairs* 30, no. 4 (2011): 581–89.

Index

Note: page numbers in *italics* refer to illustrations; those followed by "n" indicate endnotes.